# Differential Diagnoses in Surgical Pathology:
# Pancreatic and Biliary Pathology

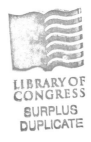

# Differential Diagnoses in Surgical Pathology:
# Pancreatic and Biliary Pathology

## Elizabeth D. Thompson, MD, PhD

Assistant Professor, Departments of Pathology and Oncology,
The Johns Hopkins University School of Medicine,
Baltimore, Maryland

## Ralph H. Hruban, MD

Baxley Professor and Director, Department of Pathology, and
the Sol Goldman Pancreatic Cancer Research Center,
The Johns Hopkins University School of Medicine,
Baltimore, Maryland

## Kiyoko Oshima, MD, PhD

Associate Professor, Department of Pathology,
The Johns Hopkins University School of Medicine,
Baltimore, Maryland

### SERIES EDITOR

## Jonathan I. Epstein, MD

Professor of Pathology, Urology and Oncology
The Reinhard Professor of Urological Pathology
Director of Surgical Pathology
The Johns Hopkins Medical Institutions
Baltimore, Maryland

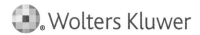

Philadelphia • Baltimore • New York • London
Buenos Aires • Hong Kong • Sydney • Tokyo

*Acquisitions Editor:* Nicole Dernoski
*Product Development Editor:* Ariel S. Winter
*Editorial Assistant:* Maribeth Wood
*Marketing Manager:* Kirsten Watrud
*Production Project Manager:* Justin Wright
*Design Coordinator:* Stephen Druding
*Manufacturing Coordinator:* Beth Welsh
*Prepress Vendor:* TNQ Technologies

9 8 7 6 5 4 3 2 1

Printed in China

**Library of Congress Cataloging-in-Publication Data**

ISBN 978-1-975144-73-9

**Cataloging in Publication data available on request from publisher**

Shop.LWW.com

# DEDICATION

*To my amazing mentors, colleagues, residents, and fellows,
who inspire me every day to be a better pathologist and teacher,
and to John, Benjamin, and Emerson, for their joyful love and support.*

Elizabeth D. Thompson

*To Claire, my wonderful and amazing wife.*

Ralph H. Hruban

*To my parents, Kimiko and Yoshio Watanabe.
I wish I could have shown them this textbook.*

Kiyoko Oshima

# PREFACE

Pathology of the pancreatobiliary tract can be an extremely challenging and treacherous area. Difficult-to-access anatomic locations often translate to small biopsy specimens where the distinction between benign, reactive processes and neoplasia can be difficult. Adding to the difficulty for pathologists is the tendency of sites like the common bile duct and ampulla to be inflamed and to demonstrate marked reactive changes secondary to both intrinsic and iatrogenic processes. Combining these changes with the presence of reactive changes surrounding mass lesions results in a plethora of neoplastic mimickers. Since the nature of samples from the pancreatobiliary tract can sometimes make ancillary studies difficult, a classic morphologic approach to differential diagnoses in this area is critical.

While larger resections may clarify some morphologic issues and allow easier integration of ancillary studies such as immunohistochemistry and molecular analyses, they present their own challenges as well. Intraductal neoplasms of the pancreas and biliary tree can be associated with extensive duct rupture and extruded stromal mucin, closely mimicking an invasive colloid carcinoma. Many solid neoplasms of the pancreas show significant morphologic overlap, such as well-differentiated neuroendocrine tumors and acinar cell carcinomas. Clear cell features can arise in a number of primary lesions in the pancreas as well as in the most commonly seen metastatic lesions, renal cell carcinoma. Luckily, there are many well-established and emerging molecular alterations, many with immunohistochemical correlates, that pathologists can call on to assist with difficult morphologic diagnoses. These include *VHL* alterations in serous cystadenomas, alterations in *CTNNB1*, the gene encoding beta catenin, in solid-pseudopapillary neoplasms, loss of Smad4 immunolabeling and diffuse p53 immunolabeling in invasive ductal adenocarcinomas, and the dichotomy of *DAXX/ATRX* alterations in well-differentiated neuroendocrine tumors with alterations in *TP53* and *Rb* in high-grade neuroendocrine carcinomas.

In this volume, we have tried to frame differential diagnostic considerations in terms of both practical morphologic considerations and layered ancillary testing, including immunohistochemistry and molecular analysis. The morphologic descriptions range from basic features to subtle distinctions that we hope will be as useful to residents in training as to practicing pathologists in various settings. Above all, we hope the differentials offered here will inspire excitement and appreciation for the interesting and challenging pathology of the pancreatobiliary tract and help us all to provide the best possible care to our patients.

**Elizabeth D. Thompson**
**Ralph H. Hruban**
**Kiyoko Oshima**

# ACKNOWLEDGMENTS

We would like to acknowledge all of our wonderful colleagues who are so generous with their time, cases, and expertise. We also thank our talented and hardworking residents and fellows whose dedication and enthusiasm for learning make the practice of pathology a joy. We are also deeply appreciative of our phenomenal pathologists' assistants and gross room staff, as our ability to diagnose difficult cases starts with a careful gross examination. Finally, we owe special thanks to Norman Barker, who lent his photographic expertise and talent to the numerous photomicrographs that illustrate this book.

# CONTENTS

Preface   vii
Acknowledgments   ix

# 1
# Pancreas

|  | Chronic Pancreatitis | Invasive Ductal Adenocarcinoma |
|---|---|---|
| *Age* | Fifth through seventh decades of life | Seventh and eighth decades of life |
| *Location* | Diffusely involves the gland | Localized, Head > tail |
| *Symptoms* | Abdominal pain radiating to the back, exocrine insufficiency with intolerance to fatty foods, and symptoms of endocrine insufficiency including glucose intolerance and eventual diabetes mellitus | Epigastric pain, painless jaundice, and nausea |
| *Signs* | Weight loss, steatorrhea, and diabetes mellitus | Weight loss and jaundice. New-onset diabetes mellitus in the elderly. 10% develop migratory thrombophlebitis |
| *Etiology* | Multiple, predominantly alcohol abuse and biliary calculi. Growing recognition of the role of germline variants in genes including *PRSS1* and *SPINK1*. Smoking contributes | Multiple, including cigarette smoking, obesity, and older age. 10% due to germline mutations in *BRCA2, BRCA1, PALB2, ATM*, p16/*CDKN2A, STK11, PRSS1*, and in DNA mismatch repair genes (*MLH1*, etc.) |
| *Histology* | 1. Lobular architecture with dense fibrosis *(Figs. 1.1.1, 1.1.3,* and *1.1.5)* <br> 2. Only rare case reports of perineural invasion by ducts, but atrophic lobules may abut nerves and benign neuroendocrine cells may be intimately associated with nerves as well *(Figs. 1.1.7* and *1.1.9)* <br> 3. No vascular invasion <br> 4. Glands separated from muscular vessels by acinar tissue, or by well-oriented connective tissue <br> 5. Area of nuclei in a single gland varies by less than 4 to 1 *(Fig. 1.1.11)* <br> 6. Lumina contain eosinophilic concretions or are empty <br> 7. Epithelial cells completely line lumina *(Fig. 1.1.13)* | 1. Haphazard growth pattern with associated desmoplasia *(Fig. 1.1.2* and *1.1.4)* <br> 2. Perineural invasion *(Fig. 1.1.8)* <br> 3. Vascular invasion *(Fig. 1.1.10)* <br> 4. Gland adjacent to a muscular vessel *(Figs. 1.1.6* and *1.1.7)* <br> 5. Area of nuclei in a single gland varies by more than 4–1 *(Figs. 1.1.12* and *1.1.15)* <br> 6. Necrotic debris in glandular lumina *(Fig. 1.1.14)* <br> 7. Incomplete lumina, with the lumina of glands directly touching stroma |
| *Special studies* | Intact Smad4 immunolabeling | Smad4 expression is lost in 55% of invasive carcinomas *(Figs. 1.1.15-1.1.18)* |
| *Treatment* | Medical, primarily supportive, including pain management, exocrine and endocrine substitution, and rarely surgery | Surgical resection for low stage disease, chemotherapy or combined chemoradiation for unresectable and locally advanced disease. Neoadjuvant therapy is becoming more common even for resectable and for borderline resectable disease |
| *Prognosis* | 50% mortality at 20–25 y post diagnosis | 9% 5-year survival |

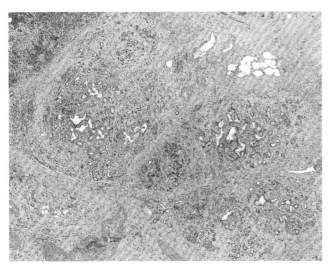

**Figure 1.1.1**    Chronic pancreatitis. Note the retention of the normal lobulated architecture, dramatic atrophy, fibrosis, and chronic inflammation.

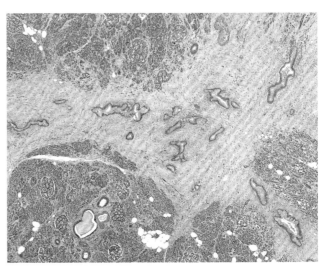

**Figure 1.1.2**    Well-differentiated invasive adenocarcinoma. Note the haphazard, infiltrative growth between lobules of pancreatic parenchyma.

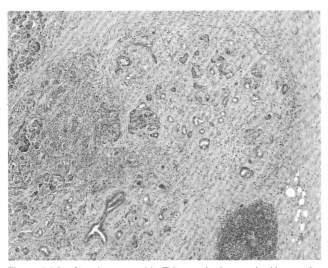

**Figure 1.1.3**    Chronic pancreatitis. This case is characterized by atrophy and associated chronic inflammation.

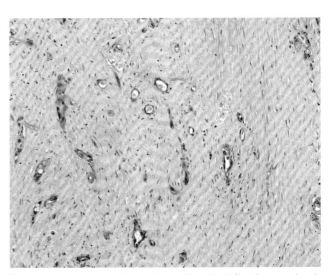

**Figure 1.1.4**    Invasive adenocarcinoma. Note the infiltrating, angulated glands in a prominent desmoplastic stroma.

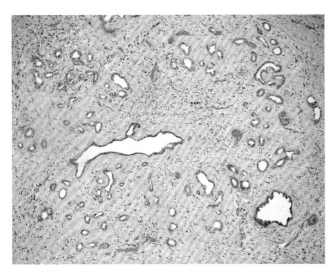

**Figure 1.1.5**    Chronic pancreatitis. Note the retained architecture and associated dense fibrosis.

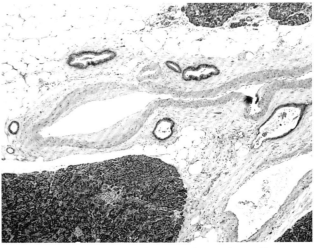

**Figure 1.1.6**    Well-differentiated invasive adenocarcinoma. The neoplastic glands are immediately adjacent to a muscular vessel.

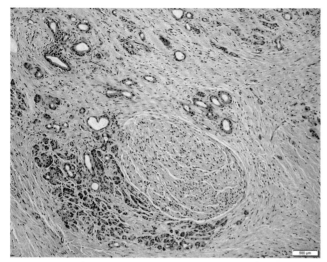

**Figure 1.1.7** Chronic pancreatitis. The acinar and ductal cells are near a nerve.

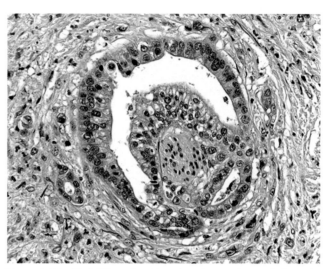

**Figure 1.1.8** Well-differentiated invasive adenocarcinoma. Perineural invasion is present.

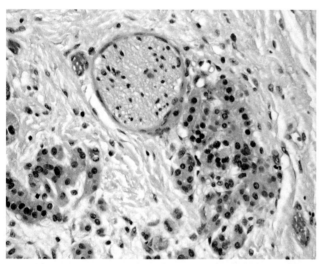

**Figure 1.1.9** Chronic pancreatitis. Nonneoplastic neuroendocrine cells are closely associated with a peripheral nerve.

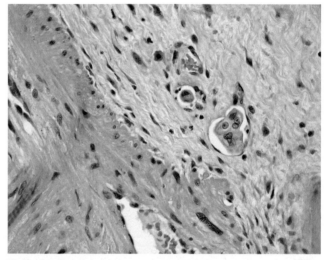

**Figure 1.1.10** Invasive ductal adenocarcinoma. Note the lymphovascular invasion.

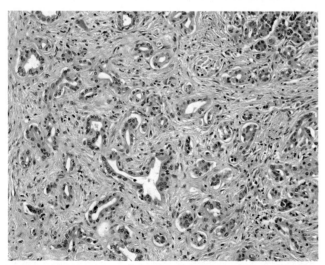

**Figure 1.1.11** Chronic pancreatitis. The nuclei are fairly uniform with only mild atypia.

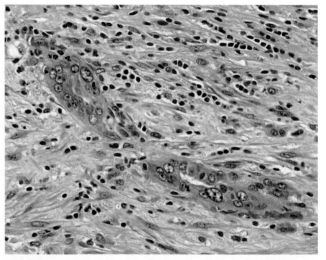

**Figure 1.1.12** Invasive ductal adenocarcinoma. Note the marked variation in nuclear size.

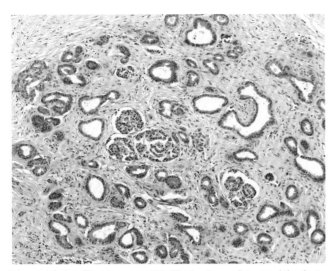

**Figure 1.1.13**   Chronic pancreatitis. The lumina are intact and the ducts atrophic.

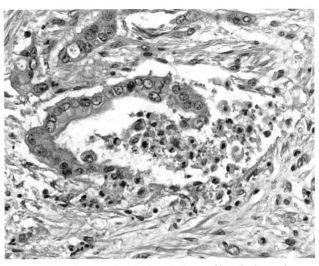

**Figure 1.1.14**   Invasive ductal adenocarcinoma. Note the incomplete lumina and luminal necrosis.

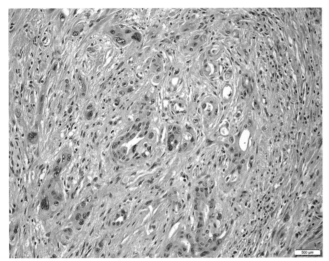

**Figure 1.1.15**   Invasive ductal adenocarcinoma. Atypical glands showing marked nuclear pleomorphism, but a vaguely lobular architecture (see corresponding Smad4 immunolabeling in Figure 1.1.16).

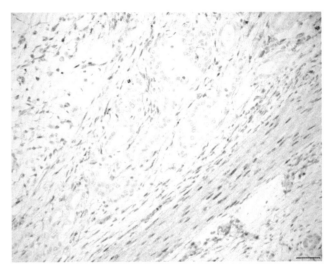

**Figure 1.1.16**   Invasive ductal adenocarcinoma. Glandular proliferation from the same case shown in Figure 1.1.15 showing loss of Smad4 labeling, confirming invasive adenocarcinoma. Note intact labeling in pancreatic stromal cells.

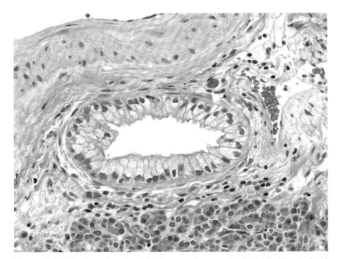

**Figure 1.1.17**   Invasive ductal adenocarcinoma. A relatively bland gland is located between pancreatic parenchyma and muscular vessel (see corresponding Smad4 immunolabeling in Figure 1.1.18).

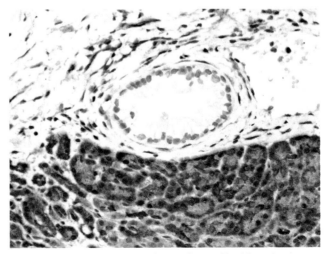

**Figure 1.1.18**   Invasive ductal adenocarcinoma. Gland from the case illustrated in Figure 1.1.17 showing loss of Smad4 labeling, confirming invasive adenocarcinoma. Note intact labeling in pancreatic parenchyma and stromal cells.

|  | Alcoholic Pancreatitis | Autoimmune Pancreatitis |
|---|---|---|
| *Age* | Fourth through seventh decades of life | Fifth and sixth decades of life |
| *Location* | Diffusely involves the gland | Often diffuse, but may be focal and mass-forming |
| *Symptoms* | Recurrent upper abdominal pain | Related to obstructive jaundice. Less often symptoms of diabetes mellitus |
| *Signs* | Steatorrhea | Jaundice, mass lesion on imaging. May have extrapancreatic autoimmune disease including sclerosing sialadenitis, sclerosing cholangitis, retroperitoneal fibrosis, and tubulointerstitial nephritis |
| *Etiology* | Alcohol abuse. Smoking can increase risk | Uncertain, but recently linked to an autoimmune reaction to a cleaved form of laminin 511 |
| *Histology* | 1. Diffuse, scattered chronic inflammation. Can see lymphoid aggregates at periphery of obstructed lobules *(Figs. 1.2.1-1.2.3)*<br>2. Inflammation associated with vasculature is not characteristic<br>3. Dense interlobular and intralobular fibrosis *(Fig. 1.2.1)*<br>4. Intraluminal laminated eosinophilic concretions and calculi *(Figs. 1.2.2-1.2.4)*<br>5. Squamous metaplasia of duct secondary to obstruction from calculi *(Fig. 1.2.4.)*<br>6. Secondary aggregation of the islets of Langerhans | 1. Duct-centric mixed inflammatory infiltrate *(Figs. 1.2.5-1.2.11)*. Lymphoid aggregates are commonly seen throughout. Type 2 has granulocytic epithelial lesions (GELs) *(Fig. 1.2.21)* (see Section 1.3)<br>2. Venulitis *(Figs. 1.2.17-1.2.20)*<br>3. Storiform fibrosis *(Figs. 1.2.13 and 1.2.15-1.2.16)*<br>4. Concretions and calculi are not characteristic<br>5. Reactive epithelial changes in duct epithelium secondary to inflammation. Neutrophils accumulate in the epithelium in the Type 2 form of the disease *(Fig. 1.2.21)*<br>6. Islet aggregation is less common but can be seen in long-standing obstructive changes secondary to mass forming autoimmune pancreatitis |
| *Special studies* | None | • Immunolabeling for IgG and IgG4 *(Figs. 1.2.12 and 1.2.14)*<br>• Type I form has increased numbers of IgG4-expressing cells (>10 cells per hpf, but typically >50 per high-power field) and increased IgG4:IgG ratio (>30%) (see Section 1.3)<br>• Special stains (VVG, Movat) can highlight elastic fibers in inflamed, damaged veins *(Figs. 1.2.18 and 1.2.20)* |
| *Treatment* | Cessation of alcohol use, pain control, replacement of exocrine and endocrine function | Immunosuppression with steroids |
| *Prognosis* | Up to a fourfold higher mortality rate compared with the general population | Excellent with treatment, some cases recur |

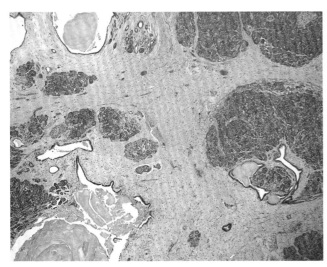

**Figure 1.2.1** Alcoholic pancreatitis. Note the dense interlobular and intralobular fibrosis with intraductal concretions. Scattered chronic inflammation.

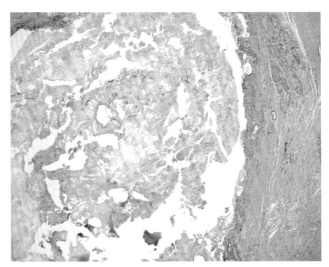

**Figure 1.2.2** Alcoholic pancreatitis. Note the characteristic eosinophilic concretions in a large duct. Scattered chronic inflammation.

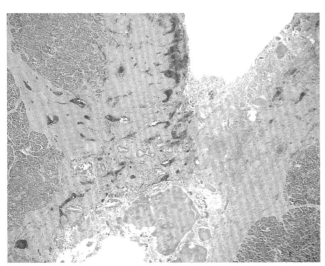

**Figure 1.2.3** Alcoholic pancreatitis. Eosinophilic concretions are associated with ruptured ducts. Scattered chronic inflammation.

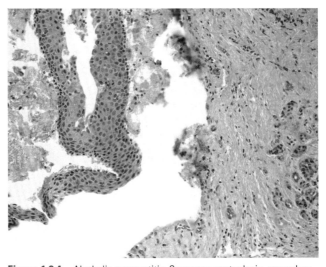

**Figure 1.2.4** Alcoholic pancreatitis. Squamous metaplasia, secondary to an intraductal calculus, involving a large duct.

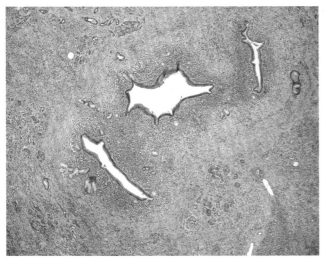

**Figure 1.2.5** Autoimmune pancreatitis. Note the duct-centric lymphoplasmacytic infiltrate in this case of Type 1 autoimmune/IgG4-related pancreatitis.

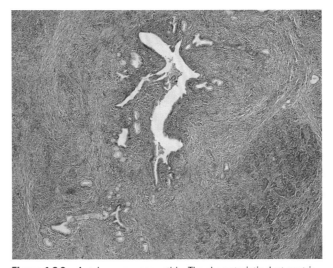

**Figure 1.2.6** Autoimmune pancreatitis. The characteristic duct-centric lymphoplasmacytic infiltrate is present.

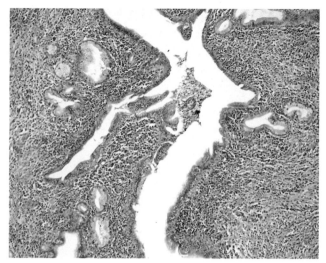

**Figure 1.2.7**    Autoimmune pancreatitis. Higher power image of the duct shown in Figure 1.2.6.

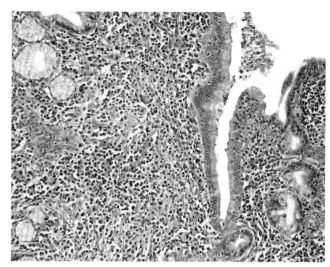

**Figure 1.2.8**    Autoimmune pancreatitis. Note the duct-centric lymphoplasmacytic infiltrate in this case of Type 1 autoimmune/IgG4-related pancreatitis.

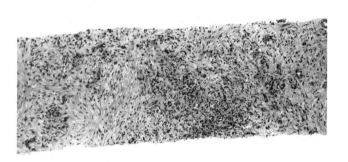

**Figure 1.2.9**    Autoimmune pancreatitis. Note the dense lymphoplasmacytic infiltrate with a suggestion of a duct-centric pattern in a biopsy of Type 1 autoimmune/IgG4-related pancreatitis.

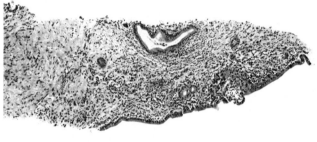

**Figure 1.2.10**    Autoimmune pancreatitis. A dense lymphoplasmacytic infiltrate is centered on a larger duct running along the edge of a biopsy in this case of Type 1 autoimmune/IgG4-related pancreatitis.

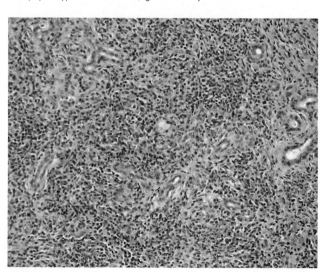

**Figure 1.2.11**    Autoimmune pancreatitis. Note the dense mixed inflammatory infiltrate.

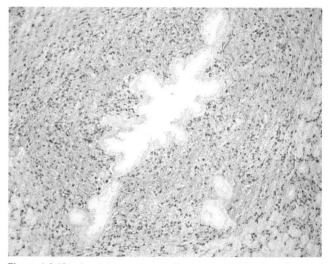

**Figure 1.2.12**    Autoimmune pancreatitis. Immunolabeling for IgG4 highlights numerous IgG4+ plasma cells.

**1.2** Alcoholic Pancreatitis vs. Autoimmune Pancreatitis    **9**

PANCREAS

1

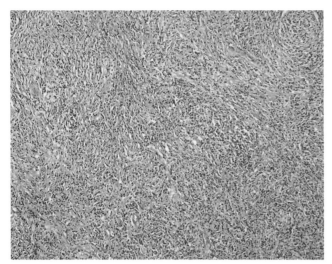

**Figure 1.2.13** Autoimmune pancreatitis. Dense mixed inflammatory infiltrate with suggestion of storiform fibrosis (see IgG4 immunolabeling in Figure 1.2.14).

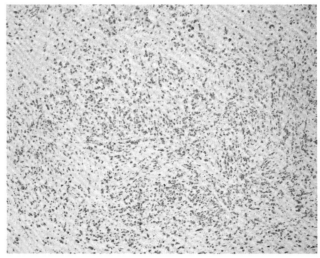

**Figure 1.2.14** Autoimmune pancreatitis. Immunolabeling for IgG4 in same case as Figure 1.2.13, highlighting numerous IgG4+ plasma cells in Type 1 autoimmune/IgG4-related pancreatitis.

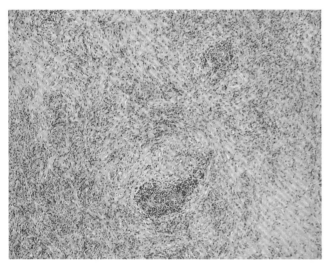

**Figure 1.2.15** Autoimmune pancreatitis. Storiform fibrosis and an associated mixed inflammatory infiltrate are present.

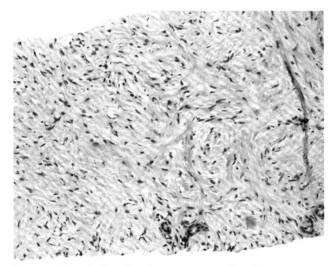

**Figure 1.2.16** Storiform fibrosis on a core biopsy from Type 1 autoimmune/IgG4-related pancreatitis.

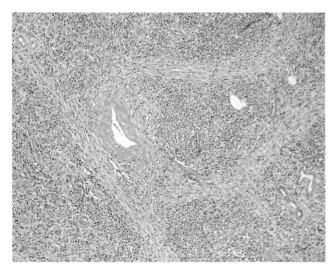

**Figure 1.2.17** Autoimmune pancreatitis. Dense inflammatory infiltrate centered on an ovoid structure adjacent to a muscular artery, consistent with venulitis (see Movat stain in Figure 1.2.18).

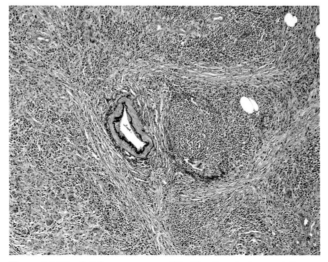

**Figure 1.2.18** Autoimmune pancreatitis. Movat pentachrome stain highlighting damaged elastic fibers in venulitis in same area shown in Figure 1.2.17.

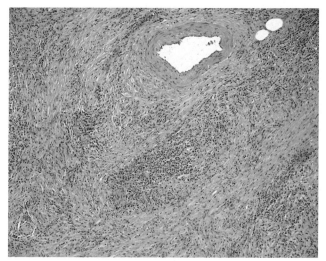

**Figure 1.2.19** Autoimmune pancreatitis. Dense inflammatory infiltrate centered on an ovoid structure adjacent to a muscular artery, consistent with venulitis (see Movat stain in Figure 1.2.20).

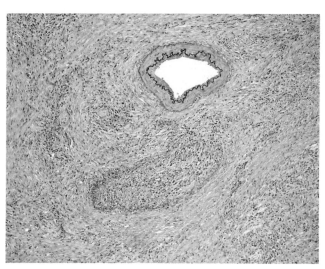

**Figure 1.2.20** Autoimmune pancreatitis. Movat pentachrome stain highlighting damaged elastic fibers in venulitis in same area shown in Figure 1.2.19.

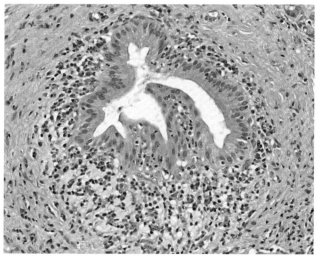

**Figure 1.2.21** Autoimmune pancreatitis. Neutrophils infiltrating duct epithelium (granulocytic epithelial lesion [GEL]) in Type 2 autoimmune pancreatitis.

# TYPE 1 (IgG4-RELATED) AUTOIMMUNE PANCREATITIS VS. TYPE 2 AUTOIMMUNE PANCREATITIS

| | Type 1 (IgG4-Related) Autoimmune Pancreatitis | Type 2 Autoimmune Pancreatitis |
|---|---|---|
| *Age* | Older, fifth and sixth decades of life | Slightly younger, fourth decade of life |
| *Location* | Often diffuse, but may be focal and mass-forming | Often diffuse |
| *Symptoms* | May cause obstructive jaundice. Less often symptoms of diabetes mellitus | Nonspecific |
| *Signs* | Jaundice, mass lesion on imaging. May have extrapancreatic autoimmune disease including sclerosing sialadenitis, sclerosing cholangitis, retroperitoneal fibrosis, and tubulointerstitial nephritis | Associated with inflammatory bowel disease |
| *Etiology* | Uncertain, but recently linked to an autoimmune reaction to a cleaved form of laminin 511 | Unknown |
| *Histology* | 1. Duct-centric mixed inflammatory infiltrate with prominent plasma cells *(Fig. 1.3.1*, see Section 1.2)<br>2. Venulitis (see Section 1.2)<br>3. Storiform fibrosis (see Section 1.2)<br>4. Neutrophils are not common | 1. Duct-centric mixed inflammatory infiltrate *(Figs. 1.3.3-1.3.8)*<br>2. Venulitis is less common<br>3. Storiform fibrosis is less common<br>4. Granulocytic epithelial lesions (GELs) characterized by collections of neutrophils within the epithelium of interlobular ducts *(Figs. 1.3.3-1.3.8)* |
| *Special studies* | • Immunolabeling for IgG and IgG4 *(Fig. 1.3.2,* see Section 1.2) reveals<br>• Increased numbers of IgG4-expressing cells (>10 cells per hpf, but typically >50 per high-power field) and increased IgG4:IgG ratio (>30%)<br>• Special stains (VVG, Movat) can highlight elastic fibers in inflamed, damaged veins (see Section 1.2) | Typically fewer (<10 per hpf) IgG4-expressing cells |
| *Treatment* | Immunosuppression | Immunosuppression |
| *Prognosis* | Excellent with treatment, more likely to recur than Type 2 | Most patients respond completely |

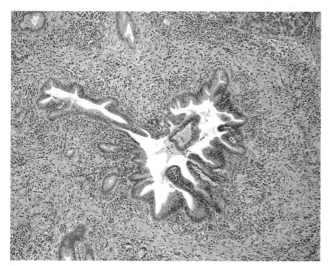

**Figure 1.3.1**   Type 1 (IgG4-related) autoimmune pancreatitis. Note the dense duct-centric lymphoplasmacytic infiltrate. See IgG4 immunostain in Figure 1.3.2.

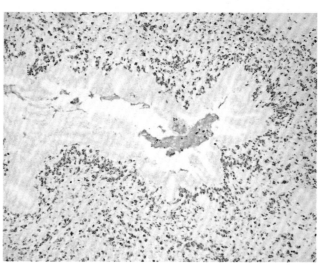

**Figure 1.3.2**   Type 1 (IgG4-related) autoimmune pancreatitis. Immunolabeling for IgG4 in the same case illustrated in Figure 1.3.1.

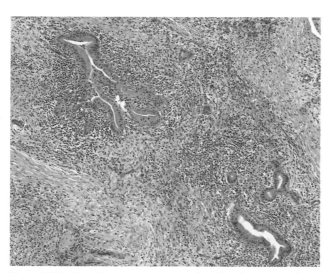

**Figure 1.3.3**   Type 2 autoimmune pancreatitis. Note the duct-centric mixed inflammatory infiltrate with pockets of neutrophils associated with ductal epithelium (granulocytic epithelial lesions [GELs]).

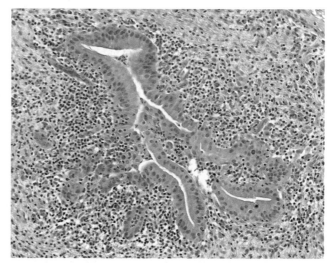

**Figure 1.3.4**   Type 2 autoimmune pancreatitis. Higher-power magnification of the case illustrated in Figure 1.3.3, highlighting GELs.

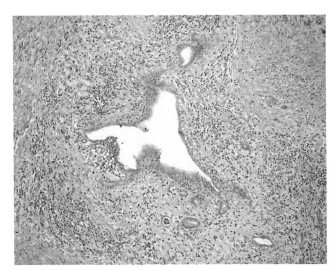

**Figure 1.3.5**  Type 2 autoimmune pancreatitis. Note the GELs.

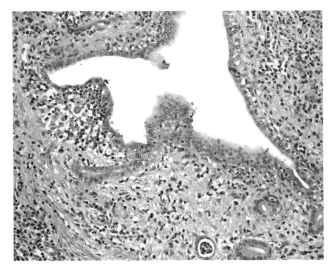

**Figure 1.3.6**  Type 2 autoimmune pancreatitis. Higher-power magnification of the case illustrated in Figure 1.3.5, highlighting GELs.

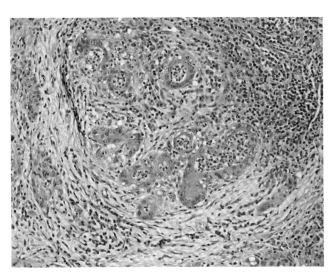

**Figure 1.3.7**  Type 2 autoimmune pancreatitis. Note the GELs.

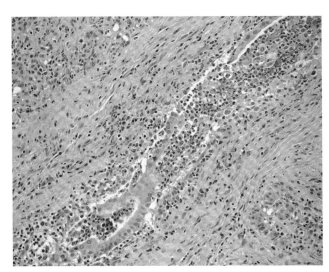

**Figure 1.3.8**  Type 2 autoimmune pancreatitis. Note the GELs.

| | Groove Pancreatitis (Paraduodenal Wall Cyst) | Inflammatory Myofibroblastic Tumor (IMT) |
|---|---|---|
| Age | Fifth through sixth decades of life | Most reports in the pancreas have been in children |
| Location | Between the head of the pancreas and the duodenum (pancreaticoduodenal groove), between the major and minor papillae | Head of pancreas |
| Symptoms | Recurrent upper abdominal pain | Pain and weight loss |
| Signs | Steatorrhea. May form mixed cystic and solid mass on imaging | Jaundice, solid mass lesion on imaging |
| Etiology | Alcohol abuse. May be caused by intraluminal concretions obstructing small ducts draining into the minor papilla | Unknown |
| Histology | 1. Cystic lesion(s) in the groove area. Cysts may contain clear fluid, necrotic material and sometimes calculi. The cysts lack an epithelial lining, or they may merge with disrupted ducts around the minor papilla *(Figs. 1.4.1-1.4.7)*<br>2. Ruptured ducts around the minor papilla<br>3. Disrupted cysts associated with myofibroblastic proliferation *(Figs. 1.4.1-1.4.7)* and more dense cellular fibrosis around the cysts may extend into the pancreas<br>4. Brunner gland hyperplasia *(Fig. 1.4.1)*<br>5. Features of alcoholic pancreatitis including eosinophilic intraductal concretions | 1. Solid, firm mass. No cystic component<br>2. No association with ducts<br>3. Spindled proliferation of myofibroblastic cells with associated marked inflammatory infiltrate (plasma cells, lymphocytes, eosinophils) *(Figs. 1.4.8-1.4.12)*<br>4. Not seen<br>5. Not seen |
| Special studies | None | • Immunolabeling with smooth muscle actin (SMA); a small subset have immunolabeling for desmin and cytokeratin<br>• Immunolabeling for anaplastic lymphoma kinase (ALK) |
| Treatment | Surgical resection, cessation of alcohol use, pain control | Complete surgical resection |
| Prognosis | Lesion is cured with resection | Limited follow-up is available for pancreas cases, but no recurrences have been reported |

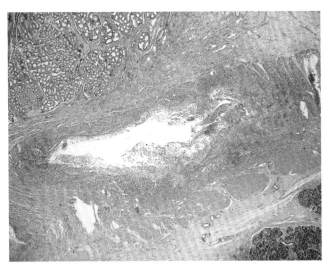

**Figure 1.4.1** Groove pancreatitis. This cystic lesion, located in the space between pancreas and duodenum, is associated with a myofibroblastic proliferation, inflammation, and Brunner gland hyperplasia (upper left).

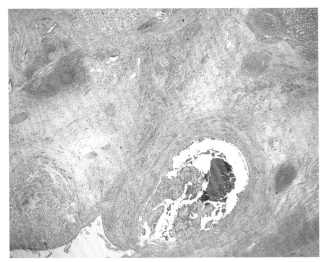

**Figure 1.4.2** Groove pancreatitis. This cystic lesion, in the space between pancreas and duodenum, is associated with myofibroblastic proliferation, inflammation, and calculi.

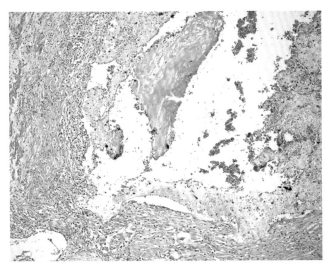

**Figure 1.4.3** Groove pancreatitis. Higher-power magnification of the case illustrated in Figure 1.4.2.

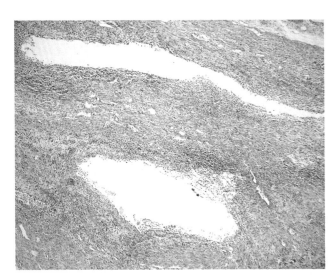

**Figure 1.4.4** Groove pancreatitis. Note the associated myofibroblastic proliferation and focal concretions. Shape of cystic lesions suggests they could represent ruptured ducts.

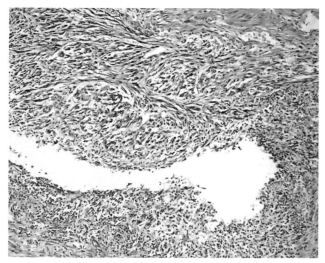

**Figure 1.4.5** Groove pancreatitis. Higher-power magnification of the case shown in Figure 1.4.4 highlights the associated myofibroblastic proliferation. Shape of cystic lesions suggests they could represent ruptured ducts.

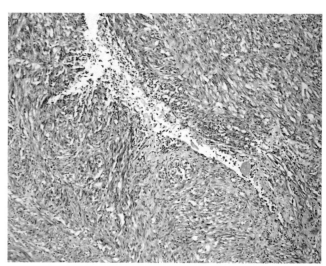

**Figure 1.4.6** Groove pancreatitis. Additional higher-power magnification of the case shown in Figure 1.4.4 highlights associated myofibroblastic proliferation. Shape of cystic lesions suggests they could represent ruptured ducts.

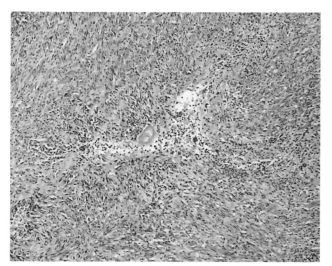

**Figure 1.4.7** Groove pancreatitis. Higher-power magnification of from the case illustrated in Figure 1.4.4. Note the associated myofibroblastic proliferation and focal concretions. Shape of cystic lesions suggests they could represent ruptured ducts.

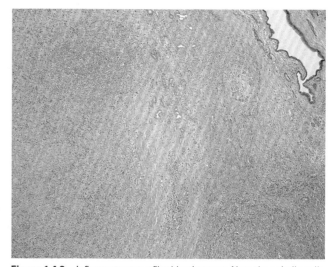

**Figure 1.4.8** Inflammatory myofibroblastic tumor. Note the spindle cells and associated mixed inflammatory infiltrate.

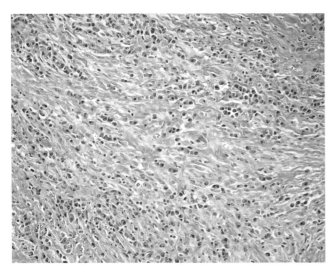

**Figure 1.4.9** Inflammatory myofibroblastic tumor. Higher-power magnification of the tumor shown in Figure 1.4.8.

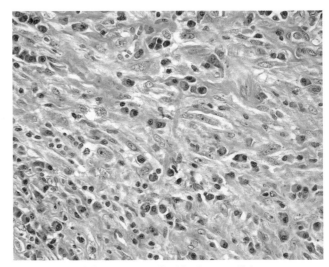

**Figure 1.4.10** Inflammatory myofibroblastic tumor. Higher-power magnification of the IMT shown in Figure 1.4.8.

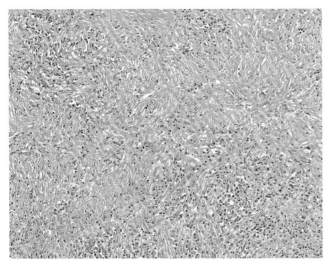

**Figure 1.4.11** Inflammatory myofibroblastic tumor.

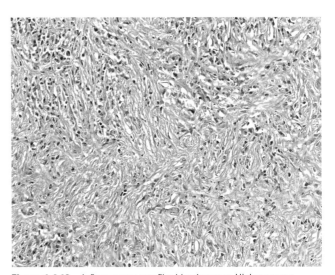

**Figure 1.4.12** Inflammatory myofibroblastic tumor. Higher-power magnification of the case shown in Figure 1.4.11.

| | Pancreatic Intraepithelial Neoplasia (PanIN) | Intraductal Papillary Mucinous Neoplasm (IPMN) |
|---|---|---|
| *Age* | Found in over half of patients >50 y of age | Mean 62–67 y of age |
| *Location* | Head > tail | Head > tail |
| *Symptoms* | Asymptomatic | Related to pancreatitis, abdominal pain |
| *Signs* | None. Not radiographically evident | Those of exocrine and endocrine insufficiency secondary to chronic pancreatitis. Radiographically evident cystic lesion |
| *Etiology* | Not known, presumably similar to invasive ductal adenocarcinoma | Not known. Small fraction have germline variants in cancer predisposition genes including *BRCA2* |
| *Histology* | 1. <5 mm. Typically not grossly evident *(Figs. 1.5.1-1.5.4)*<br>2. Usually gastric differentiation *(Figs. 1.5.1-1.5.4)*<br>3. Short papillae *(Fig. 1.5.4)* | 1. ≥1.0 cm (lesions of intermediate size [0.5–1.0 cm] may be termed "incipient IPMN"). Grossly evident *(Figs. 1.5.5 and 1.5.6)*<br>2. Neoplastic epithelium can have intestinal, gastric, or biliary differentiation *(Figs. 1.5.8-1.5.10)*<br>3. Long, well-formed, finger-like papillae *(Figs. 1.5.5-1.5.10)* |
| *Special studies* | None | Intestinal type express MUC2 and pancreatobiliary MUC1 |
| *Treatment* | None | Surgical resection based on combination of clinical, radiologic, and pathologic findings |
| *Prognosis* | Excellent. Prognosis driven by underlying pancreatic disease | Risk of synchronous and metachronous disease |

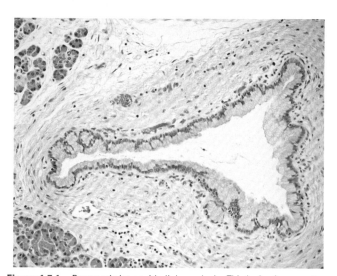

**Figure 1.5.1** Pancreatic intraepithelial neoplasia. This lesion is present in a small- to medium-sized duct and has gastric differentiation and a predominantly flat mucinous epithelium.

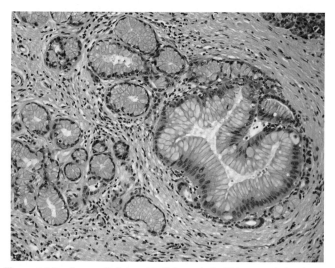

**Figure 1.5.2** Pancreatic intraepithelial neoplasia. This example involves multiple small ducts within a lobule and has gastric differentiation and a flat mucinous epithelium.

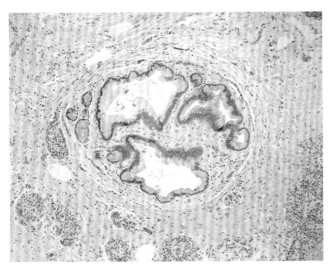

**Figure 1.5.3** Pancreatic intraepithelial neoplasia. The lesion involves multiple small ducts within a lobule and has gastric differentiation.

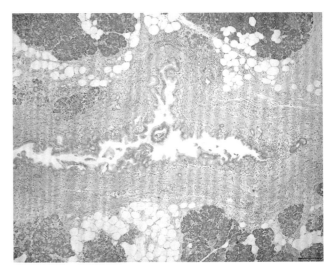

**Figure 1.5.4** Pancreatic intraepithelial neoplasia. This large PanIN lesion forms short papillary fronds.

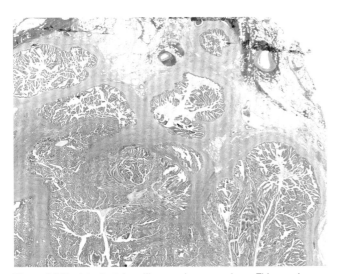

**Figure 1.5.5** Intraductal papillary mucinous neoplasm. This neoplasm extensively involves and cystically expands ducts and has a complex papillary architecture.

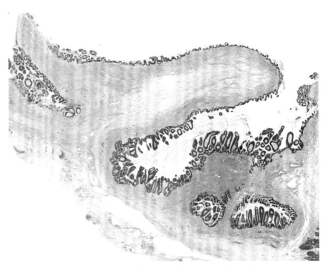

**Figure 1.5.6** Intraductal papillary mucinous neoplasm. The neoplasm involves a large duct and extends into side branch ducts. Note the intestinal differentiation.

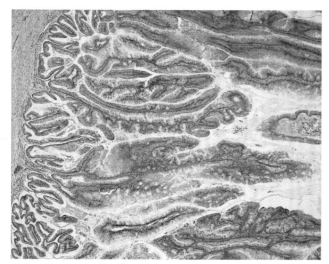

**Figure 1.5.7** Intraductal papillary mucinous neoplasm. The neoplastic epithelium forms long, well-formed, finger-like papillae.

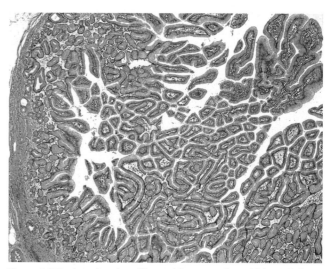

**Figure 1.5.8** Intraductal papillary mucinous neoplasm. This example has gastric differentiation. Note the long, branching papillae.

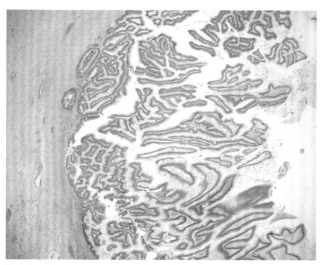

**Figure 1.5.9** Intraductal papillary mucinous neoplasm. This case has intestinal differentiation. Note the long, branching papillae.

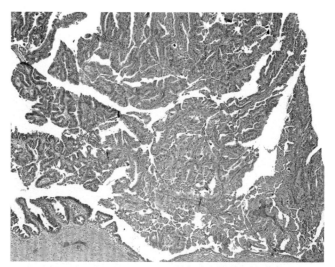

**Figure 1.5.10** Intraductal papillary mucinous neoplasm. Note the pancreatobiliary differentiation, and the long, branching, complex papillae.

|  | Pancreatic Intraepithelial Neoplasia | PanIN-like Venous Invasion |
|---|---|---|
| Age | Found in over half of patients >50 y of age | Seventh and eighth decades of life |
| Location | Head > tail | Head > tail |
| Symptoms | Asymptomatic | Those of ductal adenocarcinoma, including epigastric pain, painless jaundice, nausea |
| Signs | None | Those of ductal adenocarcinoma, including weight loss and jaundice. New-onset diabetes mellitus in the elderly |
| Etiology | Not known, presumably similar to invasive ductal adenocarcinoma | Multiple, those of ductal adenocarcinoma, including cigarette smoking, obesity, and older age. 10% due to germline mutations in *BRCA2, BRCA1, PALB2, ATM*, p16/*CDKN2A, STK11, PRSS1*, and in DNA mismatch repair genes (*MLH1*, etc.). Pancreatic ductal adenocarcinoma has a particular predilection for venous invasion |
| Histology | 1. <5 mm<br>2. Usually gastric differentiation *(Figs. 1.6.1-1.6.3)*<br>3. Short papillae or "undulating" epithelium *(Figs. 1.6.1-1.6.3)*<br>4. Involved ducts lack well-developed circumferential smooth muscle fibers *(Figs. 1.6.1-1.6.3)*<br>5. Epithelium lines the complete circumference of the involved duct *(Figs. 1.6.1-1.6.3)*<br>6. Can occur in an otherwise normal-appearing pancreas or may be associated with atrophic chronic pancreatitis *(Figs. 1.6.1-1.6.3)*<br>7. Adjacent vessels are typically open and free of fibrosis | 1. Size varies depending on vessel involved<br>2. Often pancreatobiliary differentiation *(Fig. 1.6.6)*<br>3. The epithelium is often flat, without well-developed papilla *(Figs. 1.6.5* and *1.6.6)*<br>4. Involved veins retain their appreciable circumferential smooth muscle fibers *(Figs. 1.6.4-1.6.8)*<br>5. Epithelium can completely or incompletely line the circumference of the involved vein *(Figs. 1.6.4-1.6.8)*<br>6. Pancreas contains an infiltrating ductal adenocarcinoma, and the lesions often occur at the leading edges of the carcinoma. Carcinoma within veins can sometimes appear lower grade or better differentiated than the surrounding carcinoma in the stroma *(Fig. 1.6.8)*<br>7. Adjacent vessels may have luminal fibrosis |
| Special studies | None | Stains for elastin and immunolabeling for desmin can highlight the circumferential smooth muscle fibers *(Fig. 1.6.9)* |
| Treatment | None | Same as for ductal adenocarcinoma |
| Prognosis | Excellent. Prognosis driven by underlying pancreatic disease | A poor prognostic sign. Associated with metastatic spread, particularly to the liver |

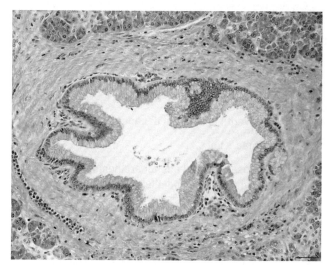

**Figure 1.6.1** Low-grade pancreatic intraepithelial neoplasia. Note the undulating epithelial surface and surrounding fibrotic stroma with rim of normal pancreatic parenchyma.

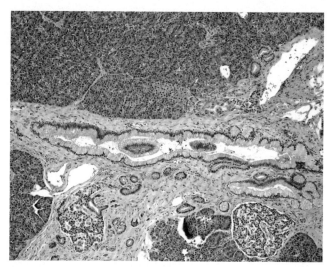

**Figure 1.6.2** Low-grade pancreatic intraepithelial neoplasia. This example involves large pancreatic ducts and forms small papillae. Note the surrounding relatively normal pancreatic parenchyma with focal atrophy.

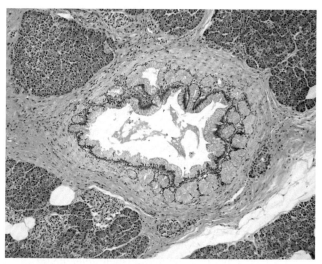

**Figure 1.6.3** Low-grade pancreatic intraepithelial neoplasia. Note the gastric-type epithelium and extension into small adjacent ducts.

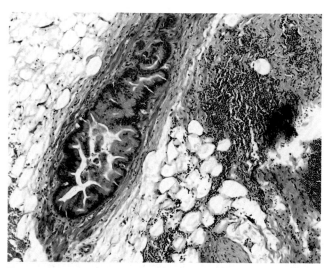

**Figure 1.6.4** Well-differentiated adenocarcinoma lining a large vein. Note the surrounding smooth muscle fibers and location centered in adipose tissue, suggesting this is the edge of the pancreas.

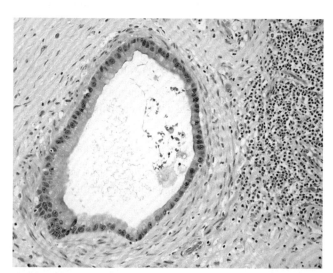

**Figure 1.6.5** Venous invasion. Note the flat epithelium, moderate atypia and pale, but well-developed surrounding smooth muscle fibers.

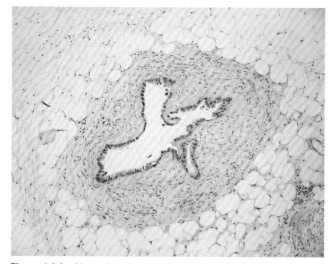

**Figure 1.6.6** Venous invasion. Note the more pancreatobiliary-type epithelium, surrounding smooth muscle fibers, and location at edge of pancreas.

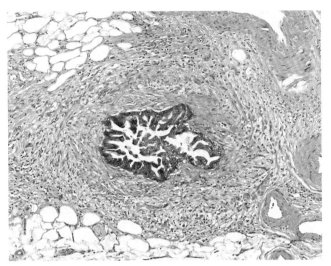

**Figure 1.6.7** Venous invasion. Note the surrounding smooth muscle fibers and location at the edge of the pancreas adjacent to other vasculature.

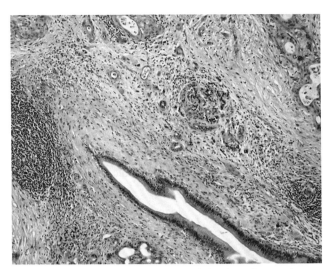

**Figure 1.6.8** Venous invasion. This example involves a larger vein. Note the surrounding invasive carcinoma and that the carcinoma within the vein has a more bland appearance (see VVG stain in Figure 1.6.9).

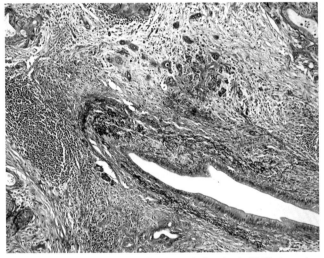

**Figure 1.6.9** Venous invasion. Special stain for elastin (VVG) shown in same area of tumor seen in Figure 1.6.8, highlighting elastic fibers in the vein wall with carcinoma lining the endothelial surface.

|  | Pancreatic Intraepithelial Neoplasia | Cancerization of Ducts |
|---|---|---|
| *Age* | Found in over half of patients >50 y of age | Seventh of eighth decades of life |
| *Location* | Head > tail | Head > tail |
| *Symptoms* | Asymptomatic | Those of ductal adenocarcinoma, including epigastric pain, painless jaundice, nausea |
| *Signs* | None | Those of ductal adenocarcinoma, including weight loss and jaundice. New-onset diabetes mellitus in the elderly |
| *Etiology* | Not known, presumably similar to invasive ductal adenocarcinoma | Multiple, those of ductal adenocarcinoma, including cigarette smoking, obesity, and older age. 10% due to germline mutations in *BRCA2, BRCA1, PALB2, ATM*, p16/*CDKN2A, STK11, PRSS1*, and in DNA mismatch repair genes (*MLH1*, etc.) |
| *Histology* | 1. <5 mm<br>2. Usually gastric differentiation *(Figs. 1.7.1 and 1.7.2)*<br>3. Short papillae *(Figs. 1.7.1 and 1.7.2)*<br>4. Gradual transitions in grade of dysplasia *(Figs. 1.7.1 and 1.7.2)*<br>5. Luminal necrosis absent<br>6. May be present in otherwise normal-appearing pancreatic parenchyma or in a background of chronic pancreatitis *(Fig. 1.7.1)* | 1. Usually <5 mm, but may involve larger ducts<br>2. Often pancreatobiliary differentiation *(Figs. 1.7.3-1.7.8)*<br>3. The epithelium is often flat. If papillary projections are present, they are irregular and poorly formed. May see micropapillary formations *(Figs. 1.7.4 and 1.7.5)*<br>4. High-grade nuclear cytology with abrupt transitions with normal ductal epithelium in a single duct *(Figs. 1.7.4-1.7.6 and 1.7.8)*<br>5. Luminal necrosis may be present *(Fig. 1.7.6)*<br>6. Often microscopically immediately adjacent to an invasive ductal adenocarcinoma *(Fig. 1.7.3)* |
| *Special studies* | None | Immunolabeling for Smad4 and TP53 will match the pattern of labeling seen in the associated invasive carcinoma *(Fig. 1.7.9)* |
| *Treatment* | None | Same as for ductal adenocarcinoma |
| *Prognosis* | Excellent. Prognosis driven by underlying pancreatic disease | Same as for ductal adenocarcinoma |

**1.7** Pancreatic Intraepithelial Neoplasia (PanIN) vs. Cancerization of the Ducts **25**

PANCREAS

1

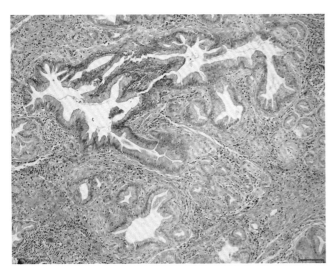

**Figure 1.7.1** Pancreatic epithelial neoplasia (PanIN). Note the smooth transition between grades of dysplasia, in a background of chronic pancreatitis.

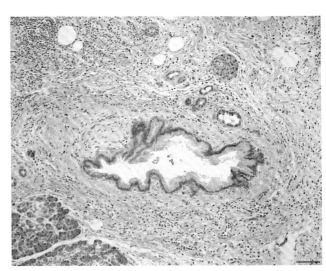

**Figure 1.7.2** Pancreatic epithelial neoplasia. The neoplastic epithelium forms short papillae and completely lines a small duct.

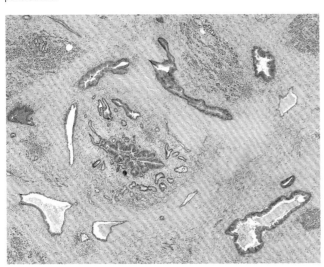

**Figure 1.7.3** Cancerization of the ducts. The invasive carcinoma has grown back into a preexisting duct native duct (cancerization). Note the adjacent invasive carcinoma in the stroma (see higher power image in Figure 1.7.4).

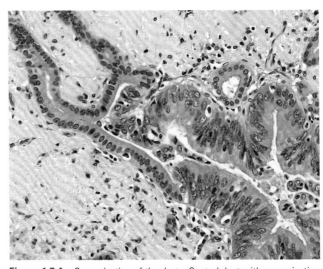

**Figure 1.7.4** Cancerization of the ducts. Central duct with cancerization from Figure 1.7.4 with abrupt transition from normal duct to high-grade epithelium.

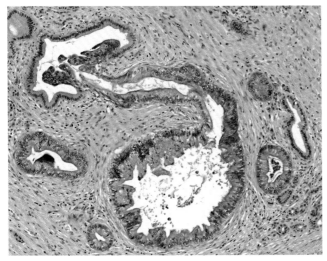

**Figure 1.7.5** Cancerization of the ducts. Note the abrupt transition from normal duct to high-grade epithelium.

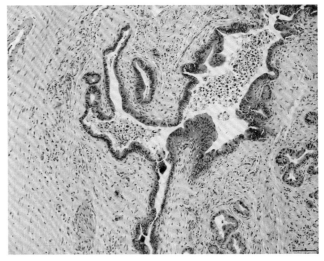

**Figure 1.7.6** Cancerization of the ducts. Carcinoma lining a native duct with abrupt transition from normal duct to high-grade epithelium. Note the luminal debris and necrosis.

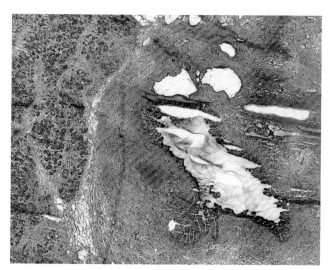

**Figure 1.7.7**    Cancerization of the ducts. This is a frozen section of a pancreatic neck margin (see higher power image in Figure 1.7.8).

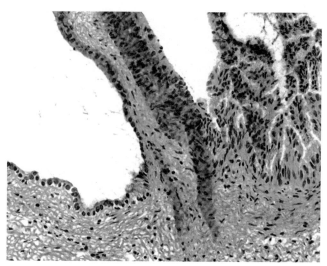

**Figure 1.7.8**    Cancerization of the ducts. Same case as shown in Figure 1.7.7. Note the abrupt transition from normal duct to high-grade epithelium.

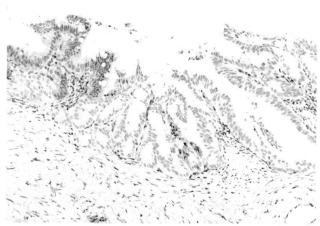

**Figure 1.7.9**    Cancerization of the ducts. Note the loss of Smad4 labeling in colonizing carcinoma with abrupt transition to intact Smad4 labeling in adjacent normal duct epithelium.

| | Intraductal Papillary Mucinous Neoplasm (IPMN) With Low-Grade Dysplasia | Intraductal Papillary Mucinous Neoplasm (IPMN) With High-Grade Dysplasia |
|---|---|---|
| Age | Mean age ~65 y | Mean age ~68 y of age |
| Location | Head > tail | Head > tail |
| Symptoms | Related to pancreatitis, abdominal pain | Related to pancreatitis, abdominal pain |
| Signs | Signs of exocrine and endocrine insufficiency secondary to chronic pancreatitis | Signs of exocrine and endocrine insufficiency secondary to chronic pancreatitis |
| Etiology | Not known. Small fraction have germline variants in cancer predisposition genes including *BRCA2* | Not known. Small fraction have germline variants in cancer predisposition genes including *BRCA2* |
| Histology | 1. ≥1 cm<br>2. May involve the main or branch pancreatic ducts, and can have a variety of directions of differentiation<br>3. Flat epithelium or well-formed papillae with fibrovascular cores<br>4. Epithelium comprised of well-oriented tall columnar mucin-containing cells<br>5. Minimal nuclear crowding, focal pseudostratification, mild nuclear enlargement, and only mild nuclear hyperchromatism *(Figs. 1.8.1-1.8.4)*<br>6. Rare mitoses. When present, mitotic figures have a normal morphology | 1. ≥1 cm<br>2. May involve the main or branch pancreatic ducts, and can have a variety of directions of differentiation<br>3. Complex architecture with papillary or micropapillary growth, fusion of papillae, and/or budding of clusters of cells into lumina. Occasionally cribriform growth *(Figs. 1.8.5-1.8.8)*<br>4. Loss of epithelial polarity with diminished mucin content *(Figs. 1.8.5-1.8.8)*<br>5. Nuclear crowding, nuclear enlargement, nuclear hyperchromasia, and nuclear pleomorphism *(Figs. 1.8.5-1.8.8)*<br>6. Mitoses can be observed, along with apoptosis and luminal necrosis *(Figs. 1.8.5-1.8.8)* |
| Special studies | None | None |
| Treatment | Some can be safely followed clinically based on constellation of clinical, radiographic and pathologic features | Surgical resection |
| Prognosis | Risk of synchronous and metachronous disease | May progress to invasive carcinoma if not resected. Risk of synchronous and metachronous disease |

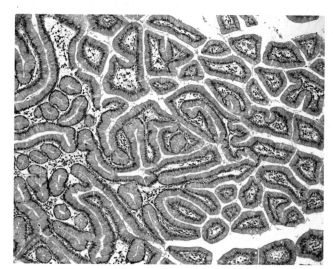

**Figure 1.8.1**    IPMN with low-grade dysplasia. The neoplasm is characterized by well-oriented, tall columnar, mucin-producing epithelium.

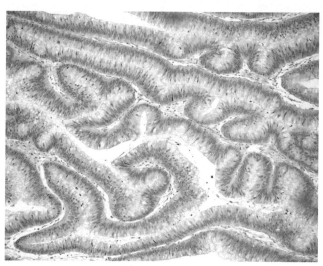

**Figure 1.8.2**    IPMN with low-grade dysplasia. The nuclei are more elongated and there is nuclear pseudostratification compared to Figure 1.8.1, but nuclei are still well oriented, and there are no complex architectural changes.

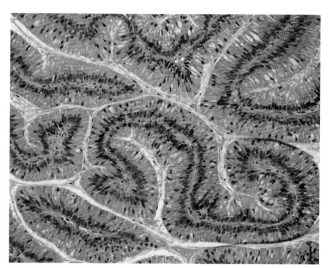

**Figure 1.8.3**    IPMN with low-grade dysplasia. Higher magnification view.

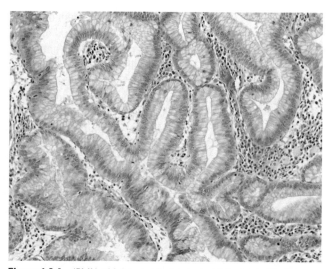

**Figure 1.8.4**    IPMN with low-grade dysplasia. Higher magnification view.

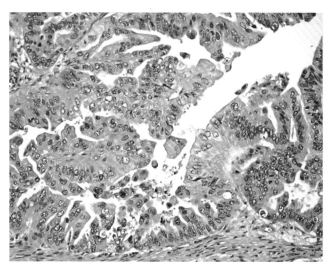

**Figure 1.8.5** IPMN with high-grade dysplasia. The neoplasm is characterized by loss of nuclear polarity, nuclear pleomorphism, enlargement and hyperchromasia, and architectural complexity (fusion of papillary fronds and micropapillary growth).

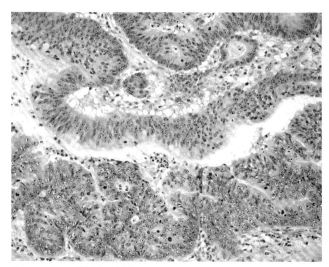

**Figure 1.8.6** IPMN with high-grade dysplasia. The neoplasm is characterized by loss of nuclear polarity, nuclear pleomorphism, numerous mitotic figures, and focal cribriform architecture.

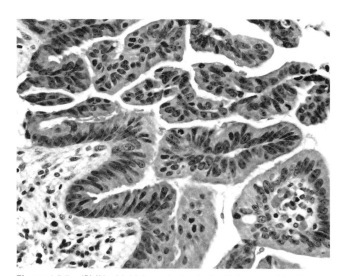

**Figure 1.8.7** IPMN with high-grade dysplasia. Higher magnification view.

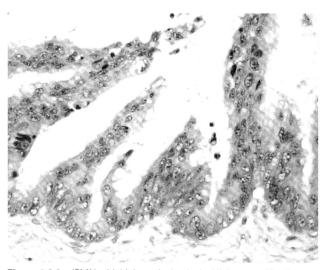

**Figure 1.8.8** IPMN with high-grade dysplasia. Higher magnification view.

**1.9**

**NONINVASIVE INTRADUCTAL PAPILLARY MUCINOUS NEOPLASM (IPMN) VS. INTRADUCTAL PAPILLARY MUCINOUS NEOPLASM (IPMN) WITH AN ASSOCIATED INVASIVE TUBULAR CARCINOMA**

| | Noninvasive Intraductal Papillary Mucinous Neoplasm (IPMN) | Intraductal Papillary Mucinous Neoplasm (IPMN) With Invasive Tubular Carcinoma |
|---|---|---|
| Age | Patients with noninvasive IPMNs are, on average, a few years younger than patients with an IPMN with an associated invasive carcinoma | Seventh and eighth decades of life |
| Location | Head > tail | Head > tail |
| Symptoms | Related to pancreatitis, abdominal pain | Related to pancreatitis, abdominal pain. Epigastric pain, painless jaundice, nausea |
| Signs | Those of exocrine and endocrine insufficiency secondary to chronic pancreatitis | Those of exocrine and endocrine insufficiency secondary to chronic pancreatitis from the IPMN. Weight loss and jaundice secondary to the invasive carcinoma. New-onset diabetes mellitus in the elderly |
| Etiology | Not known. Small percentage have germline variants in cancer predisposition genes including *BRCA2* | Not known. Small percentage have germline variants in cancer predisposition genes including *BRCA2* |
| Histology | 1. Well-defined branching pattern at low magnification as IPMN spreads through native duct system *(Figs. 1.9.1-1.9.4)*<br>2. May show any one of a variety of directions of differentiation including gastric, pancreatobiliary or intestinal, with a range of dysplasia grade<br>3. Surrounding stroma may be densely fibrotic with reactive changes associated with duct rupture<br>4. No perineural or lymphovascular invasion | 1. The glands of the invasive component deviate from a well-defined branching pattern at low magnification *(Figs. 1.9.5-1.9.10)*<br>2. Typically arise within an IPMN with high-grade dysplasia and pancreatobiliary differentiation<br>3. Infiltrative glands associated with desmoplastic response *(Figs. 1.9.9-1.9.12)*<br>4. Perineural and or lymphovascular invasion can be seen. Infiltrative glands may be seen between pancreatic lobules and adjacent to muscular vessels |
| Special studies | None | Loss of immunolabeling for Smad4 and/or diffuse immunolabeling for TP53 supports diagnosis of invasive adenocarcinoma |
| Treatment | Surgical resection according to constellation of clinical, radiologic, and pathologic features | Surgical resection with adjuvant chemotherapy |
| Prognosis | Risk of synchronous and metachronous disease | Driven by the stage of the invasive carcinoma |

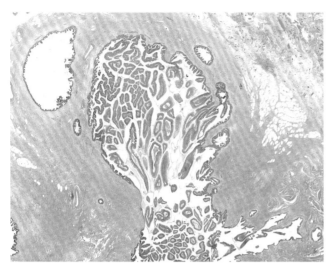

**Figure 1.9.1**    Noninvasive IPMN. Note the well-defined branching pattern with neoplastic cells confined to native duct system.

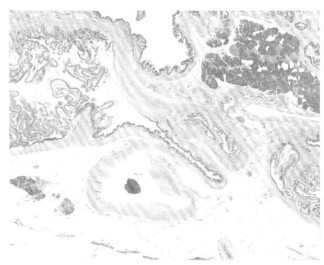

**Figure 1.9.2**    Noninvasive IPMN. Note the well-defined branching pattern and neoplastic cells confined to native duct system.

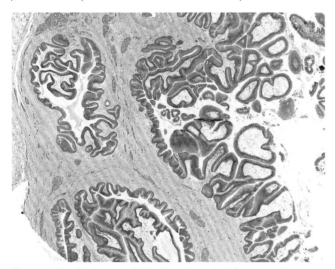

**Figure 1.9.3**    Noninvasive IPMN. Note the well-defined branching pattern and spread confined to native duct system.

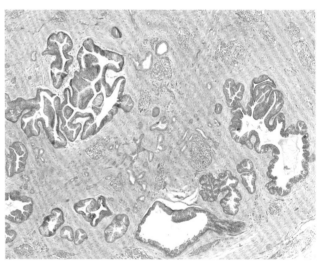

**Figure 1.9.4**    Noninvasive IPMN. Note the well-defined branching pattern and neoplastic cells confined to native duct system. Note the contrast with adjacent small ducts in atrophic lobules. IPMN focally involves small ducts but retains lobulated pattern.

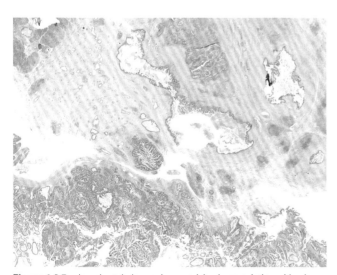

**Figure 1.9.5**    Invasive tubular carcinoma arising in association with a large IPMN. Glands of invasive adenocarcinoma are infiltrative and haphazard in their growth and contrast to the well-defined branching of the adjacent IPMN.

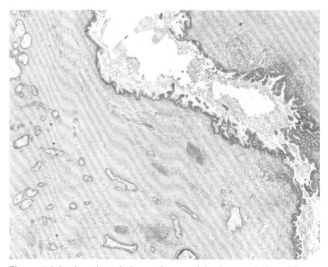

**Figure 1.9.6**    Invasive tubular carcinoma arising in association with a large IPMN. Higher-power magnification of tumor in Figure 1.9.5.

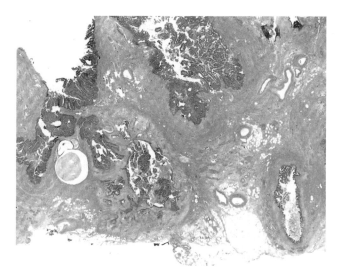

**Figure 1.9.7** Invasive tubular carcinoma arising in association with a large IPMN.

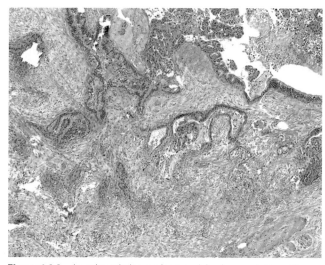

**Figure 1.9.8** Invasive tubular carcinoma arising in association with a large IPMN. Higher-power magnification of tumor in Figure 1.9.7.

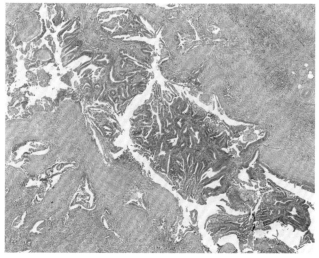

**Figure 1.9.9** Invasive tubular carcinoma arising in association with a large IPMN.

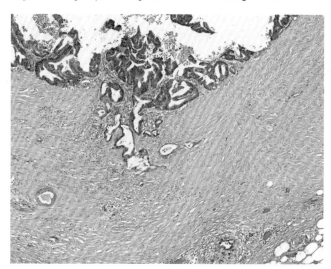

**Figure 1.9.10** Invasive tubular carcinoma arising in association with a large IPMN. The small, angulated, and irregular glands of the invasive focus are associated with desmoplastic stroma. There is a focus of perineural invasion in the bottom right quadrant.

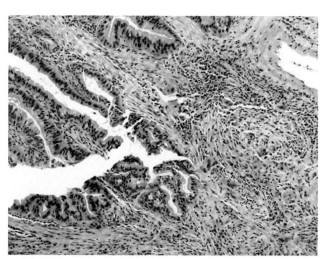

**Figure 1.9.11** Invasive tubular carcinoma arising in association with a large IPMN. Microscopic focus of invasive tubular carcinoma seen on a frozen section. This was the only focus of invasion in the case.

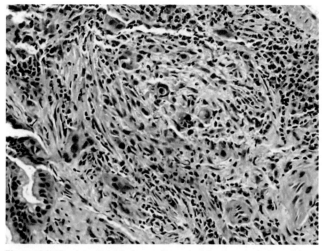

**Figure 1.9.12** Invasive tubular carcinoma arising in association with a large IPMN. Higher-power magnification on the focus of invasive carcinoma from Figure 1.9.11.

**1.10**

**INTRADUCTAL PAPILLARY MUCINOUS NEOPLASM (IPMN) WITH EXTRUDED MUCIN VS. INTRADUCTAL PAPILLARY MUCINOUS NEOPLASM (IPMN) WITH AN ASSOCIATED INVASIVE COLLOID CARCINOMA**

|  | **Intraductal Papillary Mucinous Neoplasm (IPMN) With Extruded Mucin** | **Intraductal Papillary Mucinous Neoplasm (IPMN) With Associated Invasive Colloid Carcinoma** |
|---|---|---|
| *Age* | Patients with noninvasive IPMNs are, on average, a few years younger than patients with an IPMN with an associated invasive carcinoma | Median 69–70 y |
| *Location* | Head > tail | Head > tail |
| *Symptoms* | Related to pancreatitis, abdominal pain | Related to pancreatitis, abdominal pain |
| *Signs* | Those of exocrine and endocrine insufficiency secondary to chronic pancreatitis | Those of exocrine and endocrine insufficiency secondary to chronic pancreatitis. Weight loss and jaundice |
| *Etiology* | Not known. Small fraction have germline variants in cancer predisposition genes including *BRCA2* | Not known. Small fraction have germline variants in cancer predisposition genes including *BRCA2* |
| *Histology* | 1. Intestinal-type IPMN involve native underlying duct system<br>2. Acellular pools of stromal mucin *(Figs. 1.10.1-1.10.6)*<br>3. Pools of mucin often associated with a ruptured duct *(Figs. 1.10.1-1.10.4)*<br>4. Epithelium may incompletely line duct but will retain rounded shape of underlying duct<br>5. Acellular mucin may dissect around peripheral nerves and vasculature | 1. Typically arise in association with intestinal-type IPMN *(Figs. 1.10.7-1.10.19)*<br>2. Neoplastic cells floating in pools of stromal mucin *(Figs. 1.10.7-1.10.19)*<br>3. Pools of mucin not always directly associated with a duct and dissect through stroma *(Figs. 1.10.7-1.10.19)*<br>4. Epithelium forms small clusters and irregular shapes within mucin, underlying native duct architecture is lost *(Figs. 1.10.7-1.10.19)*<br>5. May see perineural and vascular invasion by neoplastic cells *(Figs. 1.10.9, 1.10.18,* and *1.10.19)* |
| *Special studies* | None | None |
| *Treatment* | Surgical resection according to constellation of clinical, radiologic, and pathologic features | Surgical resection with adjuvant chemotherapy |
| *Prognosis* | Risk of synchronous and metachronous disease | Survival is better than for tubular ductal adenocarcinoma not arising in association with an IPMN |

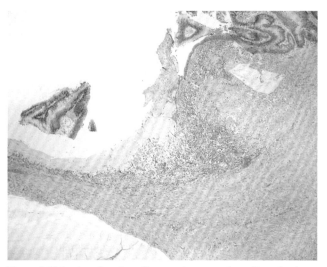

**Figure 1.10.1** Intraductal papillary mucinous neoplasm. Note the duct rupture, extruded stromal mucin, chronic inflammation and reactive stromal changes.

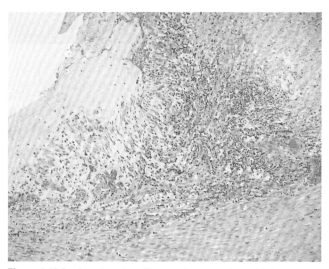

**Figure 1.10.2** Intraductal papillary mucinous neoplasm. Higher-power magnification of the case shown in Figure 1.10.1 highlighting stromal changes and inflammation in association with mucin and duct rupture.

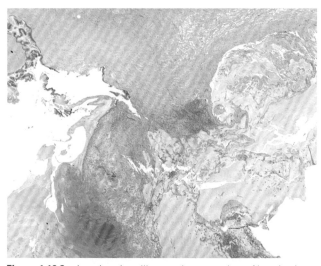

**Figure 1.10.3** Intraductal papillary mucinous neoplasm. Note the duct rupture, extensive extruded stromal mucin, chronic inflammation, and reactive stromal changes.

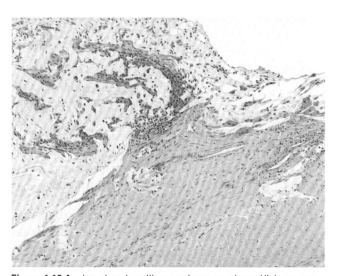

**Figure 1.10.4** Intraductal papillary mucinous neoplasm. Higher-power magnification of the case illustrated in Figure 1.10.1 highlighting extruded stromal mucin with associated chronic inflammation and giant cells, but no epithelium.

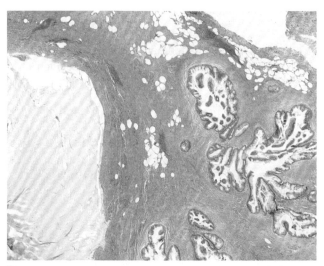

**Figure 1.10.5** Intraductal papillary mucinous neoplasm. Note the adjacent pool of acellular stromal mucin (left).

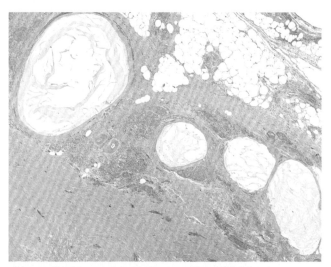

**Figure 1.10.6** Intraductal papillary mucinous neoplasm. Pools of acellular stromal mucin seen in a case of noninvasive IPMN.

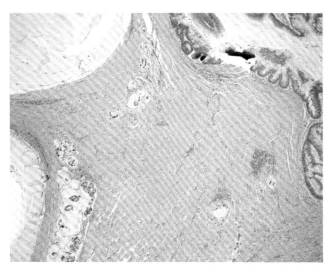

**Figure 1.10.7**  Invasive colloid carcinoma arising in association with an IPMN. Note the clusters of neoplastic epithelium floating in pools of dissected stromal mucin.

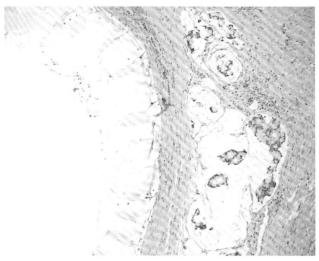

**Figure 1.10.8**  Invasive colloid carcinoma arising in association with an IPMN. Higher-power magnification of invasive colloid carcinoma shown in Figure 1.10.7.

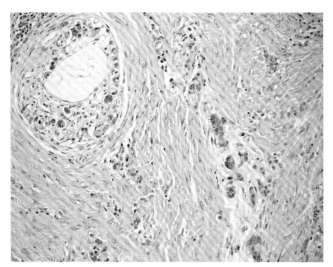

**Figure 1.10.9**  Invasive carcinoma arising in association with an IPMN. Higher-power magnification of separate area from invasive carcinoma shown in Figure 1.10.7.

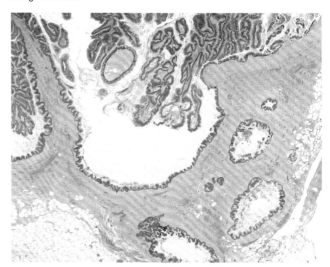

**Figure 1.10.10**  Invasive colloid carcinoma arising in association with an IPMN. Note the small focus of invasive colloid carcinoma, arising in association with the IPMN.

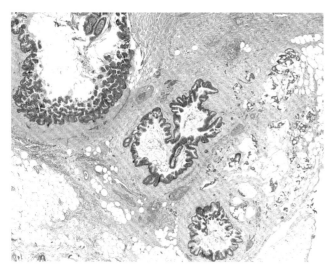

**Figure 1.10.11**  Invasive colloid carcinoma arising in association with an IPMN. Higher-magnification and deeper level of case in Figure 1.10.9. Focus of invasive colloid carcinoma expands on deeper levels.

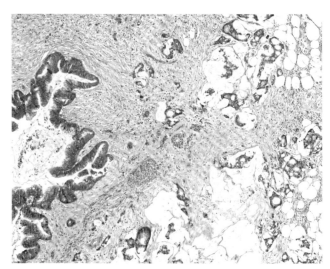

**Figure 1.10.12**  Invasive colloid carcinoma arising in association with an IPMN. Higher-magnification of invasive colloid carcinoma from Figures 1.10.9 and 1.10.10.

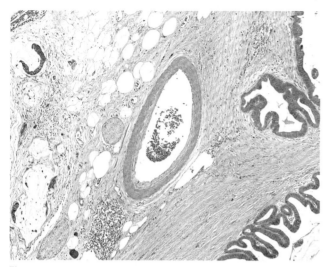

**Figure 1.10.13**    Invasive colloid carcinoma arising in association with an IPMN. Note the small focus of invasive colloid carcinoma (left).

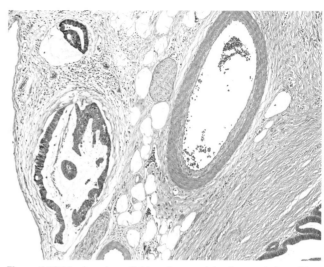

**Figure 1.10.14**    Invasive colloid carcinoma arising in association with an IPMN. Higher-magnification and deeper level of the case shown in Figure 1.10.9. Focus of invasive colloid carcinoma expands on deeper levels.

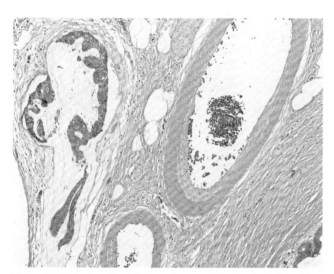

**Figure 1.10.15**    Invasive colloid carcinoma arising in association with an IPMN. Higher-magnification and deeper level of case shown in Figure 1.10.9. Focus of invasive colloid carcinoma expands on deeper levels.

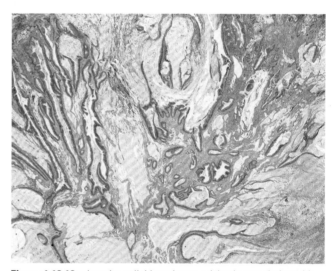

**Figure 1.10.16**    Invasive colloid carcinoma arising in association with an IPMN. The invasive colloid carcinoma is characterized by complex, dissecting pools of mucin lined by neoplastic epithelium. The mucin pools do not follow the native duct structure and neoplastic epithelium also floats within the mucin.

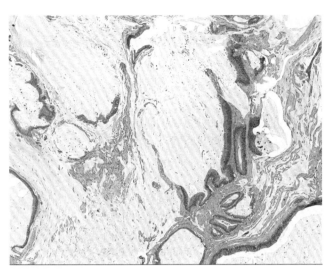

**Figure 1.10.17** Invasive colloid carcinoma arising in association with an IPMN. Higher-magnification of the invasive colloid carcinoma shown in Figure 1.10.15.

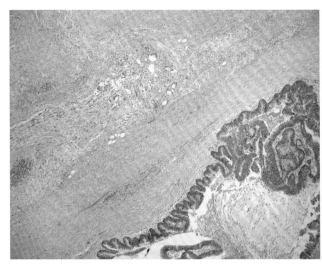

**Figure 1.10.18** Invasive carcinoma arising in association with an IPMN. Note the extensive perineural invasion.

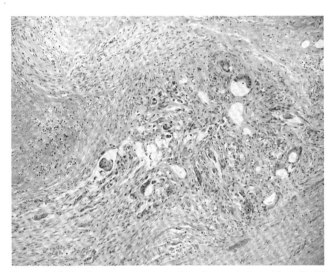

**Figure 1.10.19** Invasive carcinoma arising in association with an IPMN. Higher-magnification of invasive carcinoma shown in Figure 1.10.17.

| | Noninvasive Intraductal Papillary Mucinous Neoplasm (IPMN) | Large Duct Pattern of Invasive Adenocarcinoma |
|---|---|---|
| Age | Mean 62–67 y of age | Seventh and eighth decades of life |
| Location | Head > tail | Head > tail |
| Symptoms | Related to pancreatitis, abdominal pain | Epigastric pain, painless jaundice, nausea |
| Signs | Those of exocrine and endocrine insufficiency secondary to chronic pancreatitis | Weight loss and jaundice secondary to the invasive carcinoma. New-onset diabetes mellitus in the elderly |
| Etiology | Not known. Small percentage have germline variants in cancer predisposition genes including *BRCA2* | Likely the same as tubular adenocarcinoma |
| Histology | 1. Well-defined branching pattern at low magnification *(Figs. 1.11.1-1.11.5)*<br>2. Glands with smooth, rounded contours<br>3. Flat or well-defined papillae with fibrovascular cores<br>4. Glands confined to lobular, branching pattern of ducts, separated from muscular vessels<br>5. No perineural invasion | 1. Glands deviate from a well-defined branching pattern at low magnification. Infiltrative glands with a diameter larger than 0.5 mm or macroscopically identifiable microcysts *(Figs. 1.11.6-1.11.9)*<br>2. Glands have "jagged" contours *(Figs. 1.11.6 and 1.11.7)*<br>3. Flat epithelium, or if papillae are present they are poorly formed *(Figs. 1.11.8 and 1.11.9)*<br>4. Infiltrative lands adjacent to muscular vessels<br>5. Perineural invasion |
| Special studies | None | None |
| Treatment | Surgical resection | Surgical resection with adjuvant chemotherapy |
| Prognosis | Risk of synchronous and metachronous disease | Driven by the stage of the invasive carcinoma |

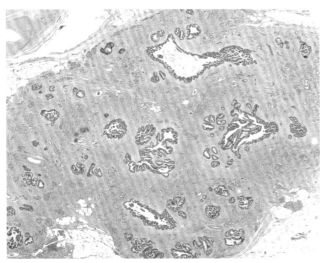

**Figure 1.11.1**    Noninvasive intraductal papillary mucinous neoplasm. This neoplasm involves the preexisting duct system. Rounded glands have a lobular configuration and well-formed papillae.

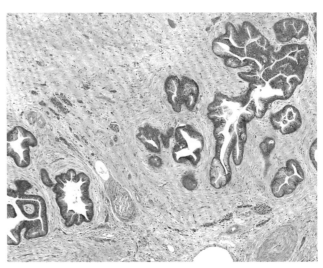

**Figure 1.11.2**    Noninvasive intraductal papillary mucinous neoplasm. Higher-magnification of the case shown in Figure 1.11.1.

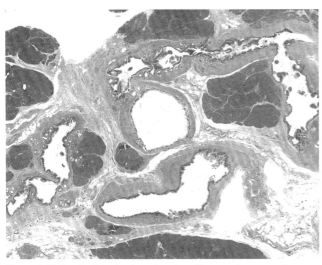

**Figure 1.11.3**    Noninvasive intraductal papillary mucinous neoplasm. This neoplasm involves large ducts.

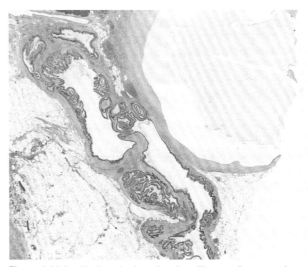

**Figure 1.11.4**    Noninvasive intraductal papillary mucinous neoplasm. This example involves large and medium-sized ducts.

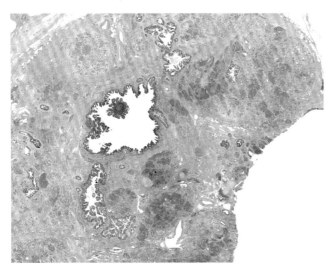

**Figure 1.11.5**    Noninvasive intraductal papillary mucinous neoplasm. This case involves large and medium-sized ducts with well-formed papillary fronds.

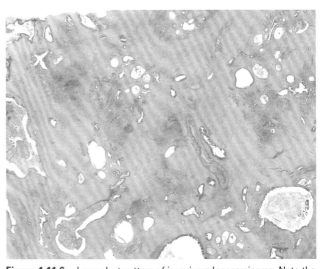

**Figure 1.11.6**    Large duct pattern of invasive adenocarcinoma. Note the infiltrative glands with "jagged" edges. Glands are not confined to the lobular configuration of the native duct system.

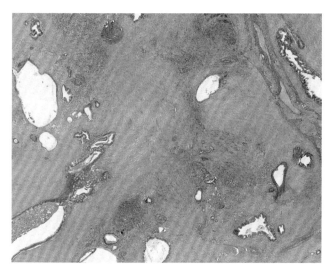

**Figure 1.11.7**   Large duct pattern of invasive adenocarcinoma. Higher magnification of the example shown in Figure 1.11.6.

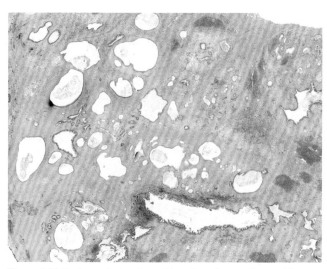

**Figure 1.11.8**   Large duct pattern of invasive adenocarcinoma. Most glands lack well-formed papillae, and many have flat epithelium.

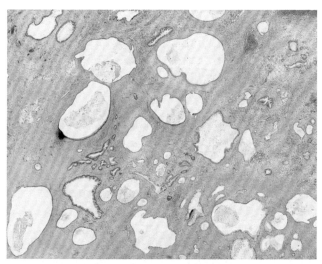

**Figure 1.11.9**   Large duct pattern of invasive adenocarcinoma. Higher-power magnification of the example shown in Figure 1.11.8.

| | Intraductal Papillary Mucinous Neoplasm (IPMN) | Intraductal Oncocytic Neoplasm (IOPN) |
|---|---|---|
| *Age* | Mean 62–67 y of age | Mean age ~60 y |
| *Location* | Head > tail | Head > tail |
| *Symptoms* | Related to pancreatitis, abdominal pain | Related to pancreatitis, abdominal pain |
| *Signs* | Those of exocrine and endocrine insufficiency secondary to chronic pancreatitis | Those of exocrine and endocrine insufficiency secondary to chronic pancreatitis |
| *Etiology* | Not known. Small percentage have germline variants in cancer predisposition genes including *BRCA2* | Not known |
| *Histology* | 1. Can have a variety of directions of differentiation, including intestinal, gastric, and pancreatobiliary *(Figs. 1.12.1 and 1.12.2)*<br>2. Flat or well-defined papillae with fibrovascular cores *(Figs. 1.12.1 and 1.12.2)*<br>3. Typically have prominent intracellular mucin *(Figs. 1.12.1 and 1.12.2)* | 1. Voluminous granular eosinophilic cytoplasm secondary to mitochondria; nuclei with single prominent nucleolus *(Figs. 1.12.5-1.12.8)*<br>2. Complex, arborizing papillae. Can form a cribriform pattern or even solid sheets *(Figs. 1.12.3-1.12.5)*<br>3. Mucin is not prominent, may have intracytoplasmic vacuoles *(Figs. 1.12.5-1.12.8)* |
| *Special studies* | • Immunolabeling parallels the direction of differentiation | • Express MUC5AC, MUC6 and 60% express HepPar-1 *(Fig. 1.12.9)*<br>• Most have a distinctive gene fusions targeting *PRKACA* or *PRKACB* |
| *Treatment* | Surgical resection | Surgical resection |
| *Prognosis* | Risk of synchronous and metachronous disease | A third of cases have an associated invasive carcinoma, usually of low stage |

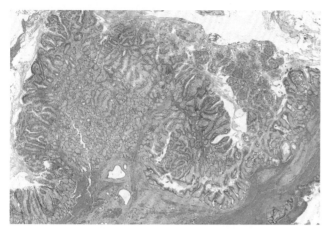

**Figure 1.12.1** Intraductal papillary mucinous neoplasm. This example has well-formed papillae with predominantly gastric differentiation and abundant intracellular mucin.

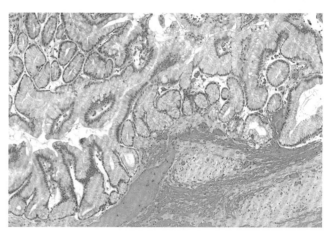

**Figure 1.12.2** Intraductal papillary mucinous neoplasm. Higher-power magnification of the case shown in Figure 1.12.1 highlighting well-formed papillae and abundant intracellular mucin.

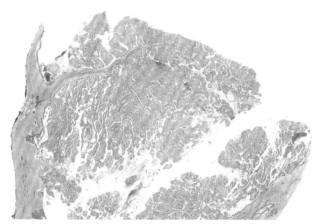

**Figure 1.12.3** Intraductal oncocytic neoplasm. Note the complex, arborizing papillae without prominent mucin.

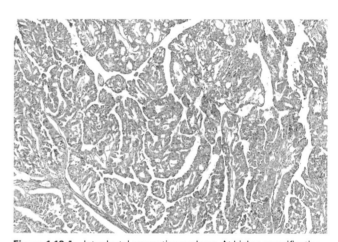

**Figure 1.12.4** Intraductal oncocytic neoplasm. At higher magnification, note the complex, arborizing papillae and focal cribriform growth.

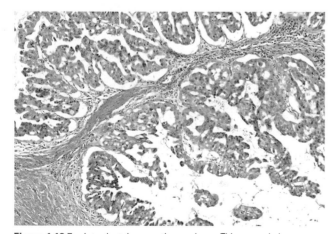

**Figure 1.12.5** Intraductal oncocytic neoplasm. This example has complex, arborizing papillae, round nuclei with single, prominent nucleoli and abundant granular, eosinophilic cytoplasm. Mucin is not prominent.

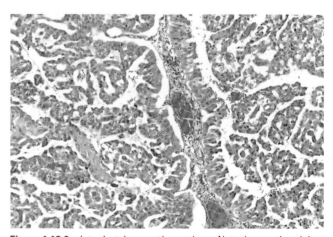

**Figure 1.12.6** Intraductal oncocytic neoplasm. Note the round nuclei with single, prominent nucleoli, and abundant granular, eosinophilic cytoplasm. Mucin is not prominent.

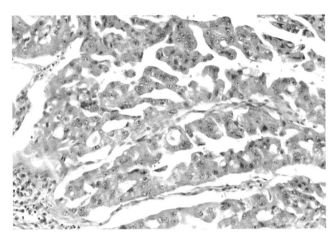

**Figure 1.12.7**   Intraductal oncocytic neoplasm. Note the round nuclei, single, prominent nucleoli, and abundant granular, eosinophilic cytoplasm. Mucin is not prominent.

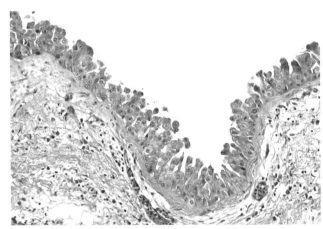

**Figure 1.12.8**   Intraductal oncocytic neoplasm. Note the round nuclei, single, prominent nucleoli, and abundant granular, eosinophilic cytoplasm. Mucin is not prominent.

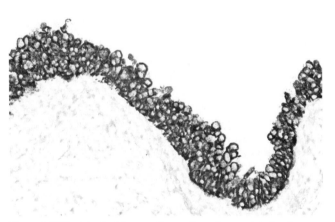

**Figure 1.12.9**   Intraductal oncocytic neoplasm. Immunolabeling for HepPar-1 in the same case as Figure 1.12.8.

| | Intraductal Papillary Mucinous Neoplasm (IPMN) | Intraductal Tubulopapillary Neoplasm (ITPN) |
|---|---|---|
| *Age* | Mean 62–67 y of age | Mean age ~55 y |
| *Location* | Head > tail | Head > tail |
| *Symptoms* | Related to pancreatitis, abdominal pain | Epigastric pain, painless jaundice, nausea |
| *Signs* | Those of exocrine and endocrine insufficiency secondary to chronic pancreatitis | Those of exocrine and endocrine insufficiency secondary to chronic pancreatitis |
| *Etiology* | Not known. Small percentage have germline variants in cancer predisposition genes including *BRCA2* | Not known |
| *Histology* | 1. Can have a variety of directions of differentiation, including intestinal, gastric and pancreatobiliary. Abundant intracellular mucin *(Figs. 1.13.1-1.13.3)*<br>2. Flat or well-defined papillae with fibrovascular cores *(Figs. 1.13.1-1.13.3)* | 1. Cuboidal cells lacking abundant mucin *(Figs. 1.13.4-1.13.12)*. Can see intracytoplasmic vacuoles or clear cell change *(Figs. 1.13.13 and 1.13.14)*<br>2. Cribriform growth pattern with tight, back-to-back glands and anastomosing papillae *(Figs. 1.13.4-1.13.14)*. Central necrosis is common (mimics ductal carcinoma in situ [DCIS] or papillary carcinoma of the breast) *(Fig. 1.13.9)* |
| *Special studies* | • Immunolabeling parallels the direction of differentiation | • Express MUC1, MUC6, and cytokeratins 7 and 19<br>• Somatic mutations are seen in chromatin remodeling genes and in the genes coding for the members of phosphatidylinositol 3-kinase (PI3K) pathway |
| *Treatment* | Surgical resection | Surgical resection |
| *Prognosis* | Risk of synchronous and metachronous disease | Almost all noninvasive cases are cured with surgical resection. 70% 5-y survival for patients with an invasive component dramatically improved relative to IPMN-associated carcinomas or ductal adenocarcinomas |

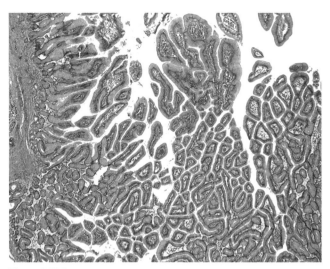

**Figure 1.13.1** Intraductal papillary mucinous neoplasm. This neoplasm forms well-defined mucinous papillary fronds.

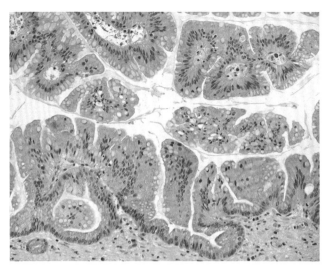

**Figure 1.13.2** Intraductal papillary mucinous neoplasm. This neoplasm has a mix of gastric and intestinal differentiation and well-defined papillae.

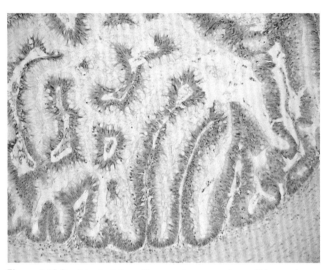

**Figure 1.13.3** Intraductal papillary mucinous neoplasm. This neoplasm has intestinal differentiation, prominent intracellular mucin, and well-defined papillae.

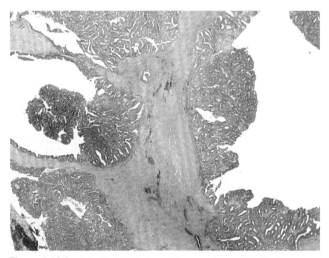

**Figure 1.13.4** Intraductal tubulopapillary neoplasm. Note the large nests of cyst-forming neoplastic cells with complex back to back glands and anastomosing papillae. Mucin is not prominent.

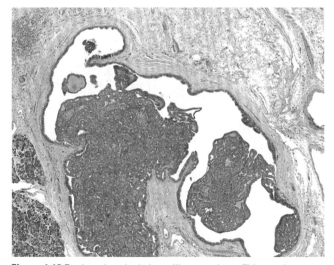

**Figure 1.13.5** Intraductal tubulopapillary neoplasm. This neoplasm forms complex back-to-back glands and anastomosing papillae.

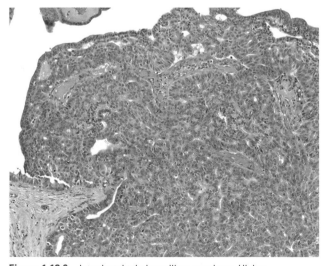

**Figure 1.13.6** Intraductal tubulopapillary neoplasm. Higher magnification of the case shown in Figure 1.13.5.

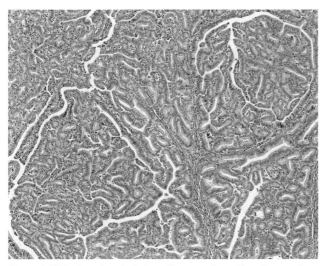

**Figure 1.13.7**    Intraductal tubulopapillary neoplasm. Note the complex back-to-back glands and anastomosing papillae.

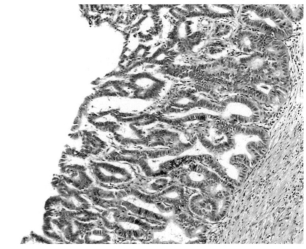

**Figure 1.13.8**    Intraductal tubulopapillary neoplasm. Note the complex back-to-back glands and anastomosing papillae.

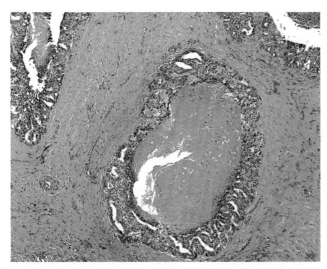

**Figure 1.13.9**    Intraductal tubulopapillary neoplasm. This case has luminal necrosis and architecture mimicking DCIS of the breast.

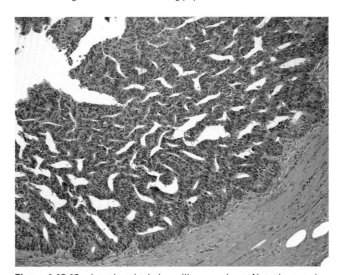

**Figure 1.13.10**    Intraductal tubulopapillary neoplasm. Note the complex back-to-back glands and anastomosing papillae. Mucin is not prominent.

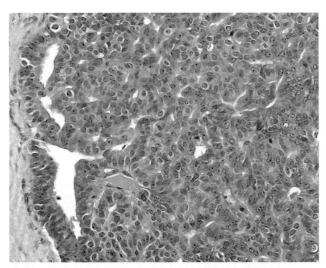

**Figure 1.13.11**    Intraductal tubulopapillary neoplasm. High magnification highlighting complex architecture and lack of prominent intracellular mucin.

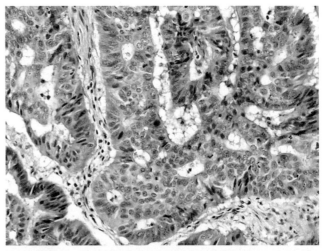

**Figure 1.13.12**    Intraductal tubulopapillary neoplasm. High magnification highlights complex architecture and lack of prominent intracellular mucin.

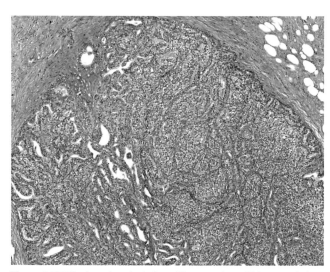

**Figure 1.13.13**    Intraductal tubulopapillary neoplasm. This example has clear cell change.

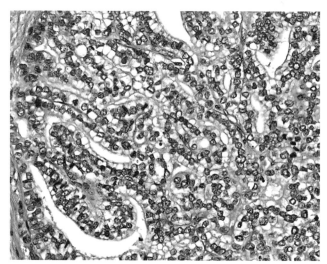

**Figure 1.13.14**    Intraductal tubulopapillary neoplasm. Higher magnification of the case shown in Figure 1.13.13, highlighting clear cell change.

| | Intraductal Tubulopapillary Neoplasm (ITPN) | Intraductal Growth of Acinar Carcinoma |
|---|---|---|
| Age | Mean age ~55 y | Mean age ~60 y |
| Location | Head > tail | Throughout the gland |
| Symptoms | Epigastric pain, painless jaundice, nausea | Nonspecific. Abdominal pain, nausea, and vomiting |
| Signs | Those of exocrine and endocrine insufficiency secondary to chronic pancreatitis | Weight loss. 15% have a syndrome of lipase hypersecretion with fat necrosis, arthralgias, and eosinophilia |
| Etiology | Not known | A minority have germline mutations in cancer predisposition genes including *BRCA2* |
| Histology | 1. Intraductal growth of cuboidal cells lacking abundant mucin. Can have intracytoplasmic vacuoles or clear cell change (see Section 1.13) *(Figs. 1.14.2-1.14.4)*<br>2. Cribriform growth pattern with tight, back-to-back glands and anastomosing papillae. Central necrosis is common (mimics ductal carcinoma in situ [DCIS] or papillary carcinoma of the breast) *(Figs. 1.14.1-1.14.4)* (see Section 1.13)<br>3. Gradual transition with adjacent epithelium<br>4. Can have intraluminal necrosis, but secretions are not prominent<br>5. Invasive carcinoma is not invariably present. Can be entirely intraductal | 1. Intraductal growth of polygonal cells with abundant granular cytoplasm and nuclei with single prominent nucleoli *(Figs. 1.14.7, 1.14.9-1.14.12)*<br>2. Sheet-like growth. Can be solid or form acini *(Figs. 1.14.7, 1.14.9-1.14.12)*<br>3. Abrupt transition to nonneoplastic ductal epithelium. Nonneoplastic epithelium typically surrounds the exophytic nodules of neoplastic cells *(Fig. 1.14.10)*<br>4. Eosinophilic intraluminal secretions<br>5. Associated invasive acinar cell carcinoma |
| Special studies | • Immunolabel for MUC1 *(Fig. 1.14.5)*, MUC6<br>• Express cytokeratins 7 and 19<br>• Somatic mutations in chromatin remodeling genes and in the genes encoding for members of the phosphatidylinositol 3-kinase (PI3K) pathway | • Immunolabel with antibodies to trypsin, chymotrypsin and Bcl10 (carboxyl ester hydrolase) *(Figs. 1.14.6 and 1.14.8)*<br>• Express cytokeratins 8 and 18<br>• Somatic *RAF* gene fusions, among others |
| Treatment | Surgical resection | Surgical resection followed by systemic chemotherapy |
| Prognosis | Almost all noninvasive cases are cured with surgical resection. 70% 5-y survival for patients with an invasive component dramatically improved relative to IPMN-associated carcinomas or ductal adenocarcinomas | Metastases may be less common than with similarly sized nonintraductal acinar cell carcinomas |

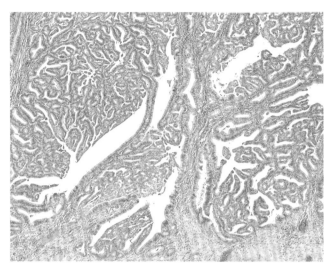

**Figure 1.14.1** Intraductal tubulopapillary neoplasm. Note the complex back-to-back tubules and anastomosing papillae.

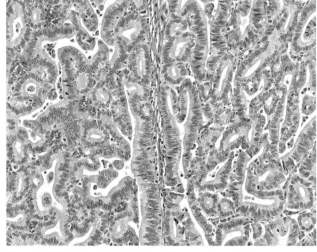

**Figure 1.14.2** Intraductal tubulopapillary neoplasm. Higher magnification of the case shown in Figure 1.14.1.

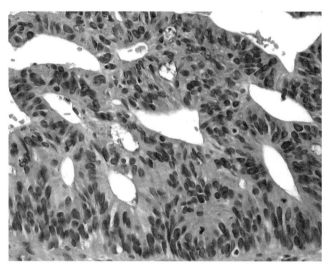

**Figure 1.14.3** Intraductal tubulopapillary neoplasm. Note the back-to-back tubules and without prominent intracellular mucin.

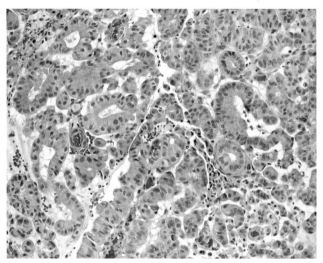

**Figure 1.14.4** Intraductal tubulopapillary neoplasm. Complex back-to-back tubules are characteristic. See MUC1 and Bcl10 immunolabeling in Figures. 1.14.5 and 1.14.6.

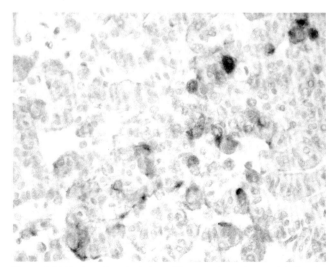

**Figure 1.14.5** Intraductal tubulopapillary neoplasm. Immunolabeling for MUC1. Same case as Figure 1.14.4.

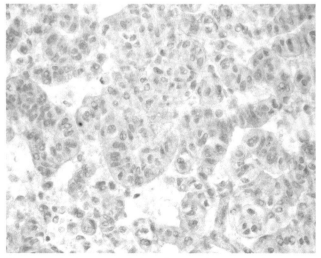

**Figure 1.14.6** Intraductal tubulopapillary neoplasm. Immunolabeling for Bcl10 is negative. This is the same case as the one shown in Figure 1.14.4.

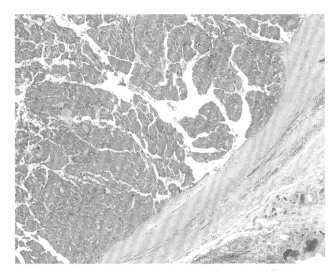

**Figure 1.14.7** Intraductal growth of acinar cell carcinoma. The neoplastic cells grow in sheets.

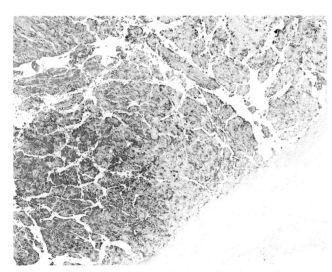

**Figure 1.14.8** Intraductal growth of acinar cell carcinoma. The neoplastic cells immunolabel with antibodies for Bcl10. This is the same case as shown in Figure 1.14.7.

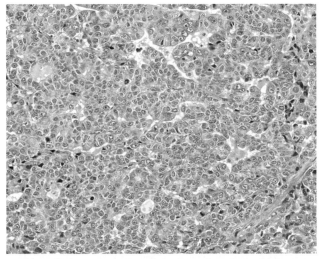

**Figure 1.14.9** Intraductal growth of acinar cell carcinoma. Higher magnification of the case shown in Figure 1.14.7 highlights acinar formation and nuclei with single prominent nucleoli.

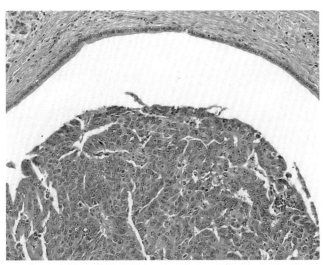

**Figure 1.14.10** Intraductal growth of acinar cell carcinoma. Note the abrupt transition to normal adjacent nonneoplastic duct epithelium.

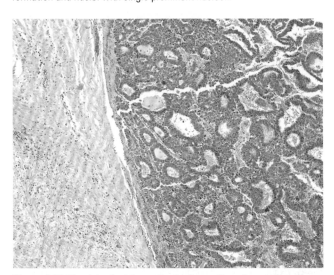

**Figure 1.14.11** Intraductal growth of acinar cell carcinoma. Note the acinar formation and prominent nucleoli.

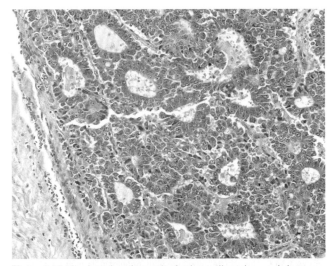

**Figure 1.14.12** Intraductal growth of acinar cell carcinoma. Acinar formation and prominent nucleoli are characteristic.

|  | Intraductal Papillary Mucinous Neoplasm (IPMN) | Mucinous Cystic Neoplasm (MCN) |
|---|---|---|
| *Age* | Mean 62–67 y of age. Slight predilection for males | Mean age ~48 y. Strong predilection for females |
| *Location* | Head > tail | Tail > head |
| *Symptoms* | Related to pancreatitis, abdominal pain | Epigastric pain, and abdominal fullness |
| *Signs* | Those of exocrine and endocrine insufficiency secondary to chronic pancreatitis | Weight loss, large abdominal mass (often discovered incidentally) |
| *Etiology* | Not known. Small percentage have germline variants in cancer predisposition genes including *BRCA2* | Not known |
| *Histology* | 1. Neoplastic cells involve and grow along the duct system<br>2. Can have a variety of directions of differentiation, including intestinal, gastric, and pancreatobiliary<br>3. Flat epithelium or well-defined papillae with fibrovascular cores *(Figs. 1.15.1-1.15.3)*<br>4. Nonspecific fibrous/collagenous stroma *(Figs. 1.15.1-1.15.3)*<br>5. May have cyst rupture with associated reactive changes and/or associated inflammation that can make stroma appear more cellular *(Figs. 1.15.4 and 1.15.5)* | 1. Neoplastic cells do not involve the duct system<br>2. Cuboidal to tall columnar mucin-producing epithelium<br>3. Flat epithelium or well-defined papillae with fibrovascular cores, often thin cores, multiseptate, with cysts within cysts (daughter cysts) *(Figs. 1.15.6 and 1.15.7)*<br>4. Characteristic ovarian-type stroma with plump spindled cells (required for the diagnosis) *(Figs. 1.15.8 and 1.15.9)*<br>5. Commonly have degenerative changes and associated epithelial denudation, which can be extensive *(Figs. 1.15.10)* |
| *Special studies* | • Immunolabeling parallels the direction of differentiation<br>• No immunolabeling for ER or PR | • Express MUC5AC (gastric-type mucin), and cytokeratins 7, 8, 18, and 19<br>• Immunolabeling for ER and PR in ovarian stroma *(Fig. 1.15.11)*. This immunolabeling can be particularly helpful in the setting of degenerative changes and epithelial denudation |
| *Treatment* | Surgical resection based on combination of clinical, radiologic, and pathologic findings | Surgical resection |
| *Prognosis* | Risk of synchronous and metachronous disease | Essentially all noninvasive mucinous cystic neoplasms are cured by complete surgical resection |

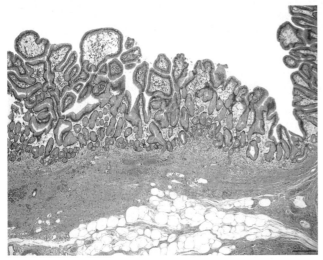

**Figure 1.15.1**    Intraductal papillary mucinous neoplasm. This case has low-grade dysplasia and dense collagenous stroma.

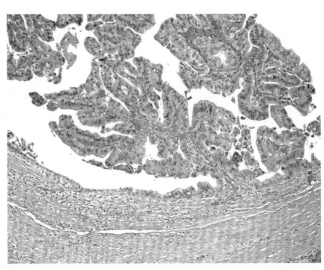

**Figure 1.15.2**    Intraductal papillary mucinous neoplasm with high-grade dysplasia. The stroma is dense and collagenous.

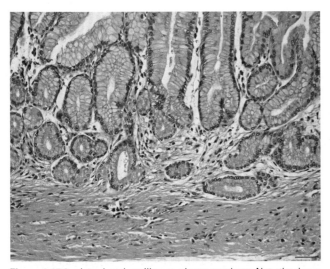

**Figure 1.15.3**    Intraductal papillary mucinous neoplasm. Note the dense collagenous stroma.

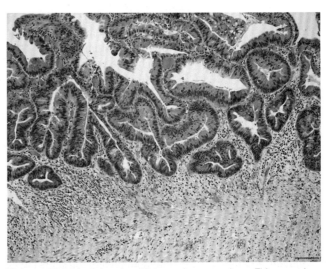

**Figure 1.15.4**    Intraductal papillary mucinous neoplasm. This example has associated inflammation creating a more cellular-appearing stroma; however, stroma remains collagenous.

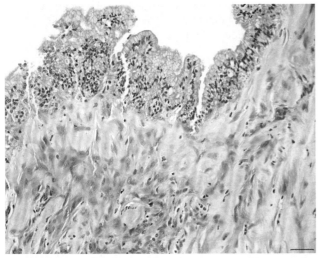

**Figure 1.15.5**    Intraductal papillary mucinous neoplasm. Note the more hyalinized stroma and reactive stromal cells consistent with prior rupture.

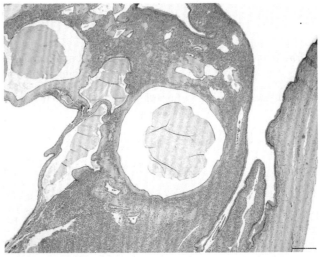

**Figure 1.15.6**    Mucinous cystic neoplasm. Note the septae, daughter cysts (cysts within cysts), and ovarian-type stroma with plump, spindled cells.

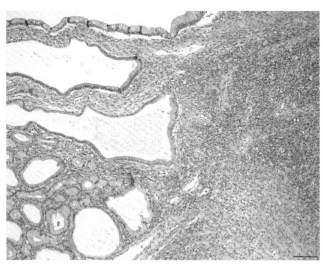

**Figure 1.15.7**　Mucinous cystic neoplasm. Note the septae, daughter cysts, and ovarian-type stroma with plump, spindled cells.

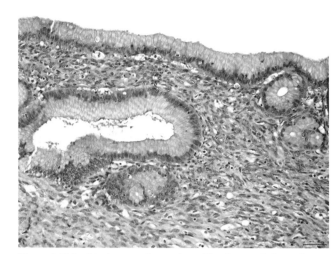

**Figure 1.15.8**　Mucinous cystic neoplasm. The characteristic ovarian-type stroma is diagnostic.

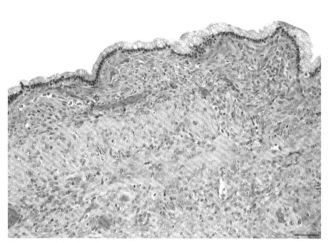

**Figure 1.15.9**　Mucinous cystic neoplasm. Note the ovarian-type stroma.

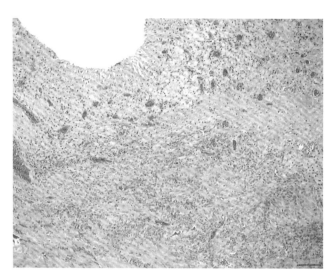

**Figure 1.15.10**　Mucinous cystic neoplasm. This case has degenerative changes and epithelial denudation. Ovarian-type stroma is still apparent beneath the eroded surface of the cyst.

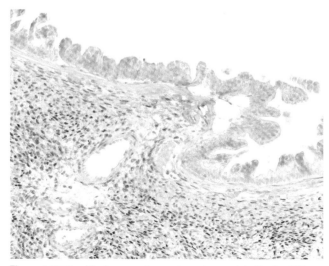

**Figure 1.15.11**　Mucinous cystic neoplasm. Immunolabeling for ER in ovarian-type stoma.

|  | Mucinous Cystic Neoplasm (MCN) | Pseudocyst |
|---|---|---|
| *Age* | Mean age ~48 y. Strong predilection for females | Adults, wide range of ages. Both sexes |
| *Location* | Tail > head | Extrapancreatic or at edge of gland |
| *Symptoms* | Epigastric pain, and abdominal fullness | Abdominal pain, anorexia |
| *Signs* | Weight loss, large abdominal mass (often discovered incidentally) | Abdominal mass after pancreatitis. Tender abdomen on examination |
| *Etiology* | Not known | Complication of acute or chronic pancreatitis. Often a strong history of alcohol abuse |
| *Gross and Histology* | 1. Cysts are intrapancreatic, but do not involve the duct system<br>2. The cyst lining is grossly smooth and often fibrotic<br>3. Cyst contents are clear mucinous or can be watery hemorrhagic<br>4. Most commonly cuboidal to columnar mucinous cyst lining, but epithelium can be attenuated with minimal mucin and/or extensively denuded *(Figs. 1.16.1-1.16.4)*<br>5. Characteristic ovarian-type stroma (required for the diagnosis). Cyst lining may be denuded with extensive inflammation, foamy macrophages, and cholesterol clefts, but ovarian-type stroma can still be identified intermixed with and beneath the degenerative changes *(Figs. 1.16.1-1.16.4)* | 1. Cysts are usually extrapancreatic or at edge of the gland<br>2. Cyst lining often grossly irregular and hemorrhagic<br>3. Cysts may contain necrotic debris<br>4. No true epithelial lining. Cyst lined by varied amounts of granulation tissue, mixed acute and chronic inflammation and, foamy macrophages. Associated fibrosis is often present *(Figs. 1.16.6-1.16.11)*<br>5. Reactive stromal change and myofibroblastic proliferation can be seen, but ovarian-type stroma is lacking *(Figs. 1.16.6 and 1.16.9)* |
| *Special studies* | • Ovarian stroma labels with antibodies to estrogen and progesterone receptors and to inhibin *(Fig. 1.16.5)*<br>• Cyst fluid with elevated CEA<br>• Molecular analysis of cyst fluid may show mutations in *KRAS, TP53*, etc | • Cyst fluid high in amylase<br>• Molecular analysis of cyst fluid negative for mutations |
| *Treatment* | Surgical resection | Medical management or drainage |
| *Prognosis* | Essentially all noninvasive mucinous cystic neoplasms are cured by surgical resection | ~5% mortality rate |

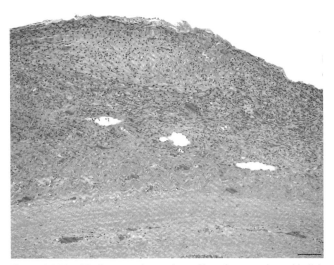

**Figure 1.16.1** Mucinous cystic neoplasm. Note the extensive epithelial denudation and associated degenerative changes. Ovarian-type stroma is apparent beneath the denuded epithelium.

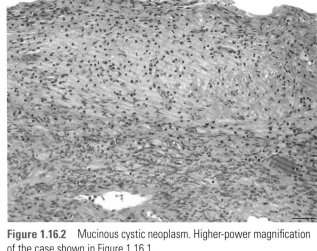

**Figure 1.16.2** Mucinous cystic neoplasm. Higher-power magnification of the case shown in Figure 1.16.1.

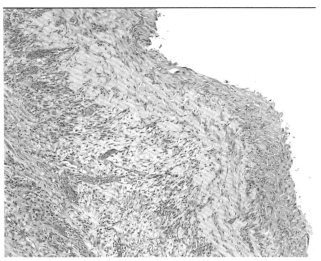

**Figure 1.16.3** Mucinous cystic neoplasm. Although there is extensive epithelial denudation, the ovarian-type stroma is apparent.

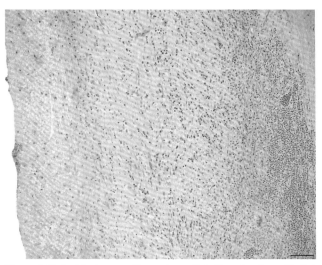

**Figure 1.16.4** Mucinous cystic neoplasm. Note the extensive epithelial denudation and associated degenerative changes. Ovarian-type stroma is apparent beneath the denuded epithelium. See immunolabeling for ER in Figure 1.16.5.

**Figure 1.16.5** Mucinous cystic neoplasm. This is the same case shown in Figure 1.16.4 with immunolabeling for ER in ovarian-type stroma present beneath epithelial denudation and degenerative changes.

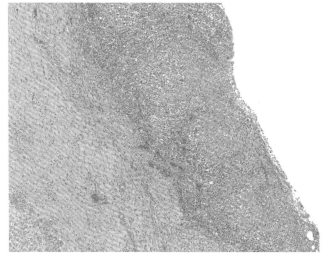

**Figure 1.16.6** Pseudocyst. Note the fibrotic wall, granulation tissue, and mixed acute and chronic inflammation. A true epithelial lining is lacking. There is reactive myofibroblastic proliferation but no organized ovarian-type stroma.

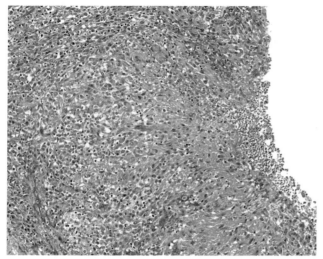

**Figure 1.16.7**   Pseudocyst. Higher-power magnification of the pseudocyst wall from Figure 1.16.6.

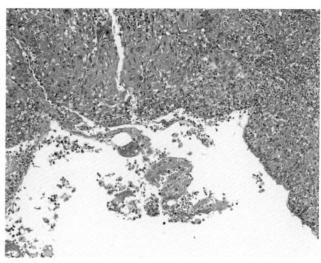

**Figure 1.16.8**   Pseudocyst. Higher-power magnification of separate area of pseudocyst wall from the case illustrated in Figure 1.16.7.

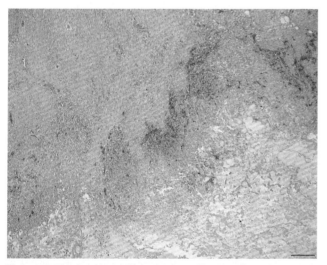

**Figure 1.16.9**   Pseudocyst. Note the dense fibrotic wall.

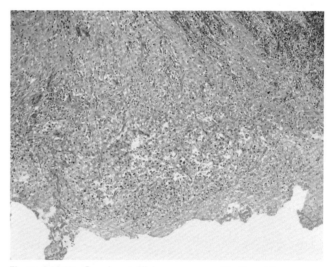

**Figure 1.16.10**   Pseudocyst. Higher-power magnification of the pseudocyst lining from Figure 1.16.9.

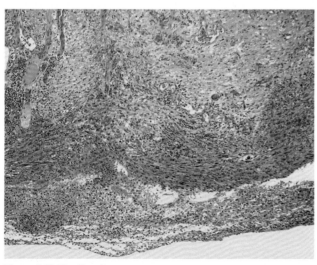

**Figure 1.16.11**   Pseudocyst.

| | Mucinous Cystic Neoplasm (MCN) With Cyst Budding | Mucinous Cystic Neoplasm (MCN) With Invasion |
|---|---|---|
| *Age* | On average, patients with noninvasive MCNs are 5 y younger than patients with an MCN with invasion. Strong predilection for females | Mean age ~48 y. Strong predilection for females |
| *Location* | Tail > head | Tail > head |
| *Symptoms* | Epigastric pain, and abdominal fullness | Epigastric pain and abdominal fullness |
| *Signs* | Weight loss, large abdominal mass (often discovered incidentally) | Weight loss, large abdominal mass (often discovered incidentally) |
| *Etiology* | Not known | Not known |
| *Histology* | 1. Cysts are intrapancreatic, but do not involve the duct system<br>2. Cysts lined by tall columnar cells with varying degrees of dysplasia<br>3. Characteristic ovarian-type stroma (required for the diagnosis)<br>4. Cells in stroma have a lobular or linear arrangement at low magnification (*Figs. 1.17.1-1.17.8*)<br>5. No reaction to the cells in the stroma. Native ducts may be entrapped in stroma (*Figs. 1.17-1.17.9-1.17.96-1.17.9*)<br>6. Neoplastic epithelial cells in stroma are similar to the clearly noninvasive component | 1. Cysts are intrapancreatic, but do not involve the duct system<br>2. Cysts lined by tall columnar cells with high-grade dysplasia<br>3. Characteristic ovarian-type stroma (required for the diagnosis)<br>4. Cells in stroma have a haphazard arrangement at low magnification (*Figs. 1.17.9-1.17.14*)<br>5. Fibrotic/desmoplastic reaction to the cells in stroma (*Figs. 1.17.10* and *1.17.12*)<br>6. Neoplastic epithelial cells in stroma may show more dramatic nuclear pleomorphism. Glands are irregular in shape (*Fig. 1.17.9*) |
| *Special studies* | None | None |
| *Treatment* | Surgical resection | Surgical resection. Possible adjuvant therapy depending on stage of the invasive component |
| *Prognosis* | Essentially all noninvasive mucinous cystic neoplasms are cured by surgical resection | Excellent, depending on stage of the invasive component. Many patients with invasion just into the ovarian-type stroma are cured |

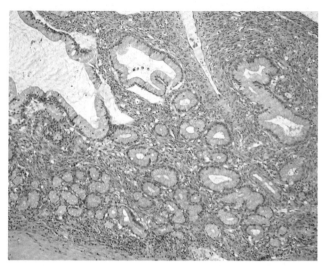

**Figure 1.17.1**    Mucinous cystic neoplasm with cyst budding. Buds are rounded and organized with in ovarian-type stroma.

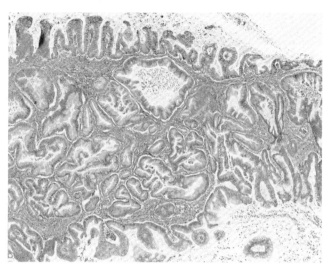

**Figure 1.17.2**    Mucinous cystic neoplasm with complex cyst budding.

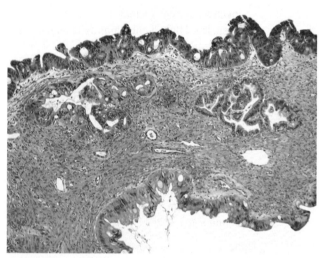

**Figure 1.17.3**    Mucinous cystic neoplasm with cyst budding. Epithelium in buds is similar to that in larger cyst, and there is no reaction to the glands within the ovarian-type stroma.

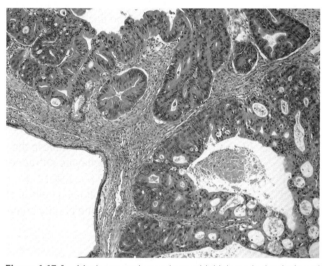

**Figure 1.17.4**    Mucinous cystic neoplasm with high-grade dysplasia and complex cyst budding.

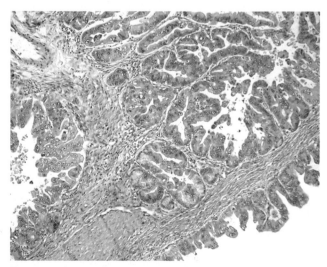

**Figure 1.17.5**    Mucinous cystic neoplasm with high-grade dysplasia and complex cyst budding.

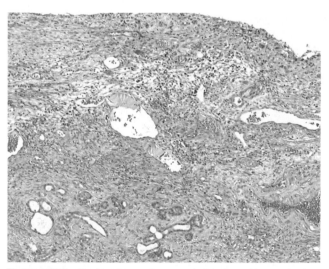

**Figure 1.17.6**    Noninvasive mucinous cystic neoplasm. Nonneoplastic ducts are entrapped within ovarian-type stroma. The ducts are lobulated and linear in configuration.

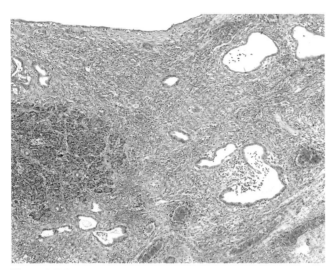

**Figure 1.17.7**    Noninvasive mucinous cystic neoplasm. Nonneoplastic ducts are entrapped within ovarian-type stroma. The ducts are lobulated in configuration.

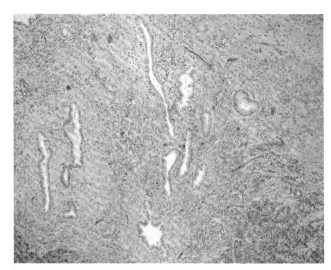

**Figure 1.17.8**    Noninvasive mucinous cystic neoplasm. Nonneoplastic ducts are entrapped within ovaria-type stroma. The ducts are lobulated and linear in configuration.

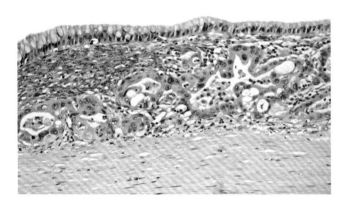

**Figure 1.17.9**    Invasive carcinoma arising in association with a mucinous cystic neoplasm. The invasive glands show an infiltrative growth pattern and dramatic nuclear pleomorphism compared to the parent cyst above.

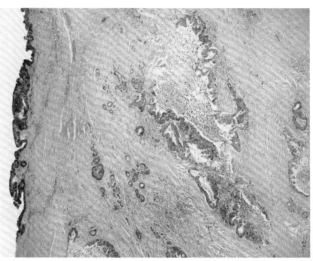

**Figure 1.17.10**    Mucinous cystic neoplasm with invasion. The invasive component has an infiltrative growth pattern in contrast to adjacent scattered, nonneoplastic ducts with a linear configuration. A desmoplastic stromal response is present.

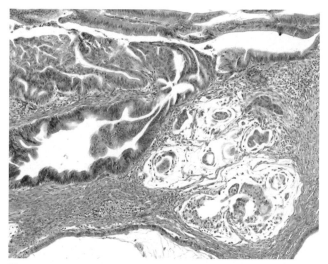

**Figure 1.17.11**    Mucinous cystic neoplasm with invasion.

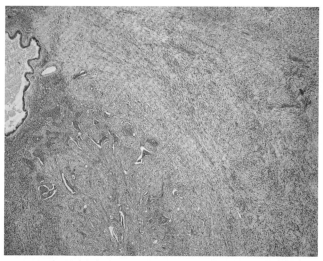

**Figure 1.17.12**    Mucinous cystic neoplasm with invasion. The invasive glands are irregular and infiltrative with a desmoplastic stromal response. An undifferentiated and spindled component is also present within the invasive carcinoma.

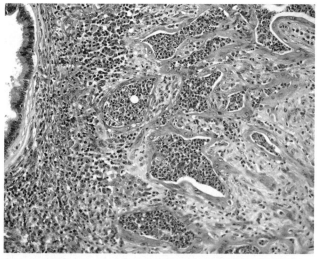

**Figure 1.17.13**    Mucinous cystic neoplasm with invasion. Higher magnification of the glandular component in the invasive carcinoma from the same case as Figure 1.17.12.

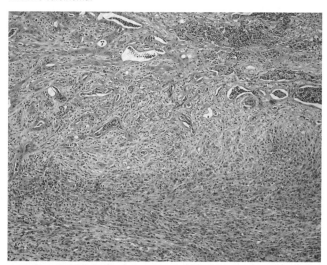

**Figure 1.17.14**    Mucinous cystic neoplasm with invasion. Higher magnification of the glandular and undifferentiated components in the invasive carcinoma from the case shown in Figure 1.17.12 (see cytokeratin AE1/3 immunolabeling in Figure 1.17.15).

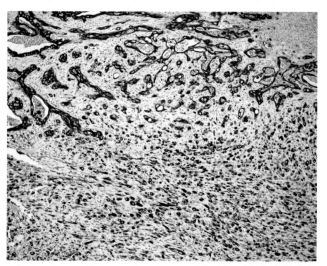

**Figure 1.17.15**    Mucinous cystic neoplasm with invasion. This is the same case as Figure 1.17.14 with immunolabeling for cytokeratin AE1/3 in both the glandular and undifferentiated components of the invasive carcinoma.

| | **Solid Serous Adenoma** | **Metastatic Renal Cell Carcinoma (RCC), Clear Cell Type** |
|---|---|---|
| *Age* | Mean age of 65 y | Mean age of 65 y |
| *Location* | Anywhere in the gland | Anywhere in the gland, typically multifocal lesions |
| *Symptoms* | Often asymptomatic. Can cause abdominal pain, early satiety, dyspepsia, weight loss, and nausea and vomiting | Most are asymptomatic. May have weight loss, abdominal pain, nausea, and vomiting |
| *Signs* | Solid mass imaging | History of renal cell carcinoma. Multifocal lesions on imaging |
| *Etiology* | Can be seen in patients with von Hippel-Lindau syndrome | Can be seen in patients with von Hippel-Lindau syndrome |
| *Histology* | 1. Cuboidal cells with optically clear cytoplasm *(Figs. 1.18.1-1.18.4)*<br>2. Solid nests or sheets of cells, often with microscopic tubules and cysts *(Figs. 1.18.1-1.18.4)*<br>3. Round, very uniform nuclei, centrally placed *(Figs. 1.18.2 and 1.18.3)* | 1. Polygonal cells with abundant clear to pale, eosinophilic cytoplasm *(Figs. 1.18.6-1.18.8 and 1.18.10)*<br>2. Sheets or small nests of cells without lumen formation and invested with delicate capillaries. Bleeding and hemosiderin are common *(Figs. 1.18.6-1.18.8)*<br>3. Slightly eccentric nuclei with more pleomorphism. Nucleoli vary with grade and can be prominent *(Fig. 1.18.8)* |
| *Special studies* | • Periodic acid Schiff (PAS) positive, sensitive to digestion (PAS-D) *(Fig. 1.18.5)*<br>• Immunolabel for cytokeratins 7, 8, 18, and 19 | • Immunolabel with antibodies for Pax8 *(Fig. 1.18.9)*<br>• Negative for cytokeratin 7 |
| *Treatment* | Surgical resection if symptomatic or if approaching important anatomic structures | Surgical resection if clinically possible, often in the absence of other metastatic disease |
| *Prognosis* | Excellent. There are benign lesions | Average survival ~5 y after surgical resection |

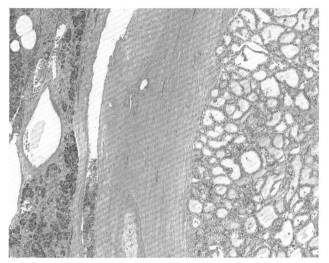

**Figure 1.18.1**  Solid serous adenoma. Note the formation of microscopic lumen.

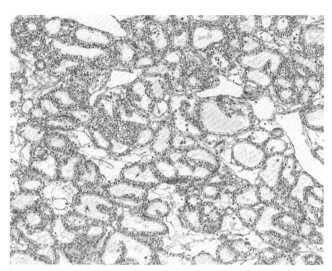

**Figure 1.18.2**  Solid serous adenoma. Higher magnification from the case shown in Figure 1.18.1. Note the optically clear cytoplasm and round, uniform, and centrally placed nuclei.

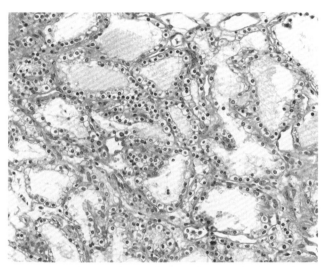

**Figure 1.18.3**  Solid serous adenoma. Additional higher magnification of the case shown in Figure 1.18.1.

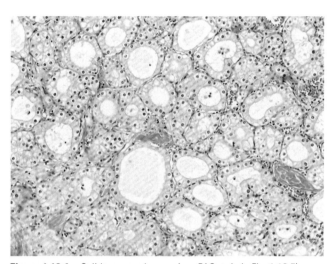

**Figure 1.18.4**  Solid serous adenoma (see PAS stain in Fig. 1.18.5).

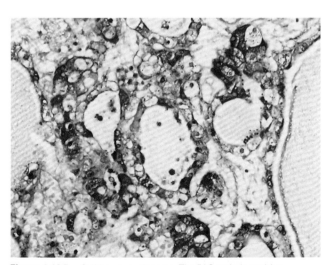

**Figure 1.18.5**  Solid serous adenoma. The PAS stain is positive.

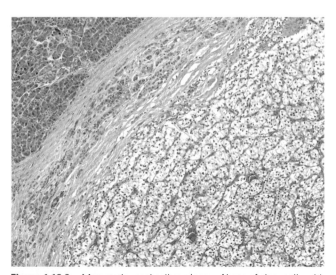

**Figure 1.18.6**  Metastatic renal cell carcinoma. Nests of clear cells with eccentric nuclei surrounded by delicate capillaries.

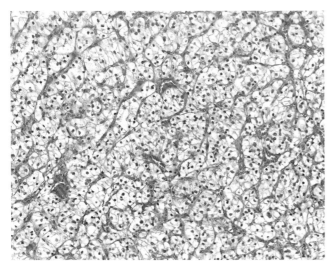

**Figure 1.18.7**    Metastatic renal cell carcinoma. Higher magnification of the case illustrated in Figure 1.18.6.

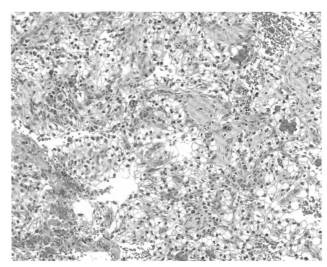

**Figure 1.18.8**    Metastatic renal cell carcinoma. Higher magnification of a separate area from same metastatic RCC shown in Figures 1.18.6 and 1.18.7. There are focal hemosiderin-laden macrophages and nuclear pleomorphism with scattered nucleoli.

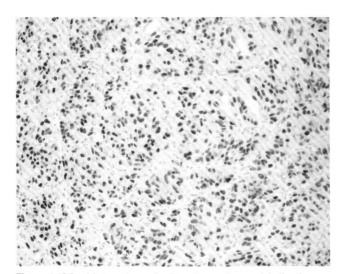

**Figure 1.18.9**    Metastatic renal cell carcinoma. Immunolabeling for PAX8 is positive.

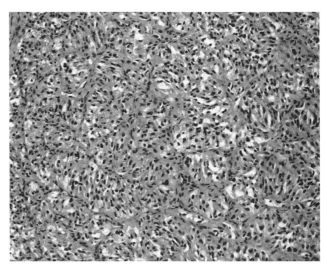

**Figure 1.18.10**    Metastatic renal cell carcinoma. This example has more eosinophilic cytoplasm.

| | Solid Serous Adenoma | PanNET with Clear Cell Change |
|---|---|---|
| *Age* | Mean age of 65 y | Most between 40 and 65 y, with a mean age of 58 y |
| *Location* | Anywhere in the gland | Throughout the gland |
| *Symptoms* | Often asymptomatic. Can cause abdominal pain, early satiety, dyspepsia, weight loss, and nausea and vomiting | Usually nonspecific, including abdominal pain and nausea |
| *Signs* | Solid mass on imaging | Solid mass on imaging with vascularity and peripheral enhancement |
| *Etiology* | Can be seen in patients with von Hippel-Lindau syndrome | Can be seen in patients with multiple endocrine neoplasia (MEN), von Hippel-Lindau syndrome, etc. |
| *Histology* | 1. Cuboidal cells with optically clear cytoplasm *(Figs. 1.19.1-1.19.5)*<br>2. Solid nests or sheets of cells, often with microscopic tubules and cysts *(Figs. 1.19.1-1.19.5)*<br>3. Round, very uniform nuclei, centrally placed *(Figs. 1.19.3-1.19.4)* | 1. Abundant foamy cytoplasm with numerous clear vesicles *(Figs. 1.19.6-1.19.9)*<br>2. Neoplastic cells form nests and cords. Cells are separated by thin-walled vessels, and there is often hemorrhage *(Figs. 1.19.6-1.19.9)*<br>3. Uniform nuclei with "salt and pepper" chromatin *(Figs. 1.19.6 and 1.19.9)* |
| *Special studies* | • Periodic acid Schiff positive, sensitive to digestion (PAS-D) (see Section 1.18)<br>• Do not express synaptophysin and chromogranin<br>• Diffusely immunolabel with antibodies to cytokeratins 7, 8, 18, and 19 | • Periodic acid Schiff positive, sensitive to digestion (PAS-D)<br>• Diffusely immunolabel with antibodies to synaptophysin and chromogranin<br>• Diffusely immunolabel with antibodies to cytokeratins 8 and 18 |
| *Treatment* | Surgical resection if symptomatic or if approaching important anatomic structures | Surgical resection when possible |
| *Prognosis* | Excellent. These are benign lesions | These are malignant tumors. Prognosis depends on grade (proliferation rate) and stage |

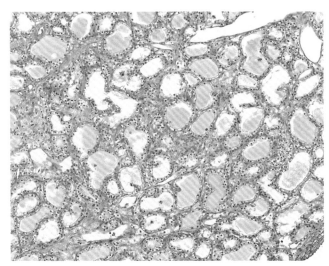

**Figure 1.19.1**    Solid serous adenoma. Note the microscopic cysts, optically clear cytoplasm and uniform, centrally placed nuclei.

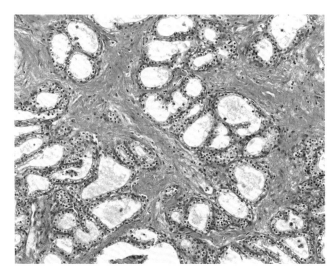

**Figure 1.19.2**    Solid serous adenoma.

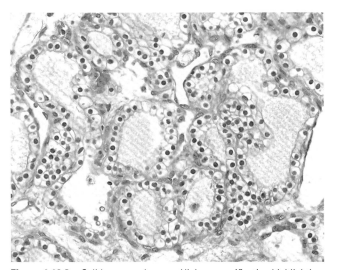

**Figure 1.19.3**    Solid serous adenoma. Higher magnification highlighting the optically clear cytoplasm and uniform, centrally placed nuclei.

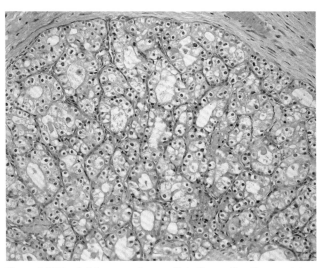

**Figure 1.19.4**    Solid serous adenoma. Note the small, uniform nuclei.

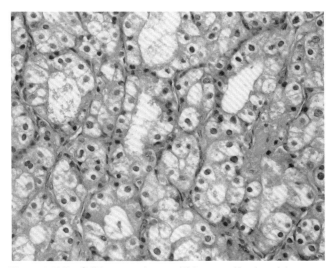

**Figure 1.19.5**    Solid serous adenoma. Higher magnification of the neoplasm shown in Figure 1.19.4.

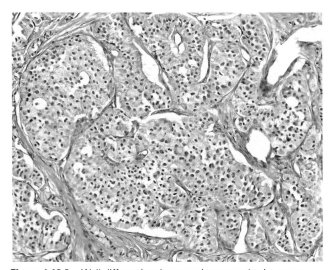

**Figure 1.19.6**    Well-differentiated pancreatic neuroendocrine tumor. Note the nests of cells with clear to foamy cytoplasm and round to oval nuclei with "salt and pepper" chromatin.

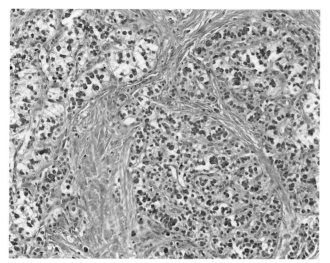

**Figure 1.19.7**    Well-differentiated pancreatic neuroendocrine tumor. The neoplastic cells form nests and cords and have clear to foamy cytoplasm.

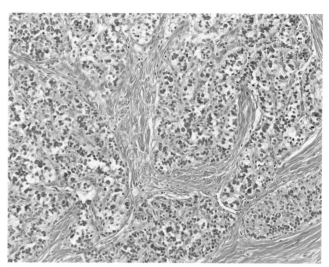

**Figure 1.19.8**    Well-differentiated pancreatic neuroendocrine tumor. Note the nests of cells with clear to foamy cytoplasm.

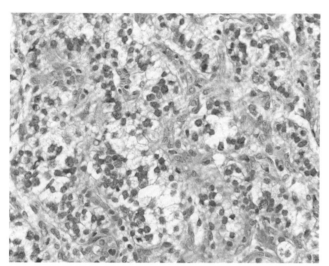

**Figure 1.19.9**    Well-differentiated pancreatic neuroendocrine tumor. Higher magnification of the case shown in Figure 1.19.8, highlights the clear to foamy cytoplasm and "salt and pepper" chromatin.

| | Acinar Cystic Transformation/Acinar Cell Cystadenoma | Serous Cystadenoma |
|---|---|---|
| *Age* | Range 18–60 y (mean age of 45 y) | Mean age of 65 y |
| *Location* | Head > tail | Anywhere in the gland |
| *Symptoms* | Usually asymptomatic | Often asymptomatic. Can cause abdominal pain, early satiety, dyspepsia, weight loss, and nausea and vomiting |
| *Signs* | Multilocular or unilocular cystic lesion on imaging | Multilocular or microcystic mass; may see central scar with sunburst calcification pattern |
| *Etiology* | Not known | Can be seen in patients with von Hippel-Lindau syndrome |
| *Histology* | 1. Cysts lined by a one- to two-cell thick layer of pyramidal cells *(Figs. 1.20.1-1.20.4, 1.20.6, and 1.20.7)*<br>2. Pyramidal cells with polarized granular cytoplasm *(Figs. 1.20.1-1.20.4, 1.20.6, and 1.20.7)*<br>3. Round nuclei with single prominent nucleoli *(Figs. 1.20.1-1.20.4, 1.20.6, and 1.20.7)*<br>4. Fine needle aspiration (FNA) often nondiagnostic because cyst lining looks like normal non-neoplastic acinar cells<br>5. Broad papillary projections are common, but small and complex papillae are uncommon | 1. Cells form microscopic cysts with clear lumina *(Figs. 1.20.8-1.20.10)*<br>2. Cuboidal cells with optically clear cytoplasm *(Figs. 1.20.9 and 1.20.10)*<br>3. Round, very uniform nuclei *(Figs. 1.20.9 and 1.20.10)*<br>4. Infarction and degenerative changes are common, particularly after fine needle aspiration *(Figs. 1.20.11 and 1.20.12)*<br>5. Complex papillae can be seen *(Figs. 1.20.13 and 1.20.14)* |
| *Special studies* | • Immunolabel with antibodies to trypsin, chymotrypsin and Bcl10 (carboxyl ester hydrolase) *(Fig. 1.20.5)*<br>• Immunolabel with antibodies to cytokeratins 8 and 18 | • Periodic acid Schiff positive (PAS) *(Fig. 1.20.15)*, sensitive to digestion (PAS-D)<br>• Immunolabel with antibodies to cytokeratins 7, 8, 18, and 19 |
| *Treatment* | Observation, but they are often resected because they clinically mimic other lesions in the pancreas | Surgical resection if symptomatic or if approaching important anatomic structures |
| *Prognosis* | Entirely benign, probably not neoplastic | Excellent. These are benign lesions |

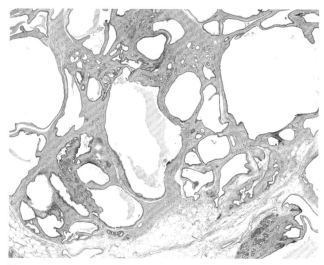

**Figure 1.20.1**    Acinar cystic transformation. Note the multiloculated cystic architecture with flat epithelium.

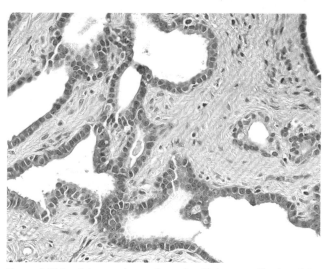

**Figure 1.20.2**    Acinar cystic transformation. Higher magnification of the cysts in Figure 1.20.1, highlighting pyramidal cells with polarized granular cytoplasm and round nuclei with single prominent nucleoli.

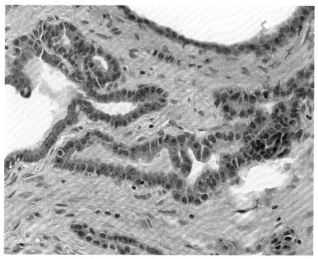

**Figure 1.20.3**    Acinar cystic transformation. Higher magnification of the cysts in Figure 1.20.1, highlighting pyramidal cells with polarized granular cytoplasm and round nuclei with single prominent nucleoli.

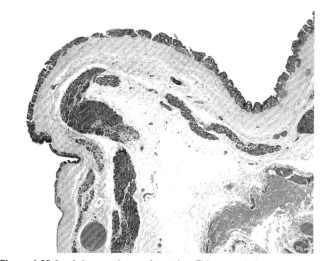

**Figure 1.20.4**    Acinar cystic transformation. This example has a unilocular cystic architecture (see immunolabeling for Bcl10 in Figure 1.20.5).

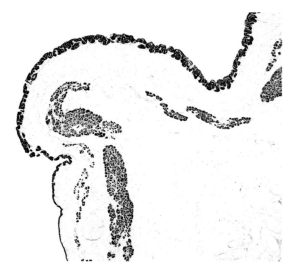

**Figure 1.20.5**    Acinar cystic transformation. Positive immunolabeling with antibodies to Bcl10 (the antibody cross reacts with carboxyl ester hydrolase).

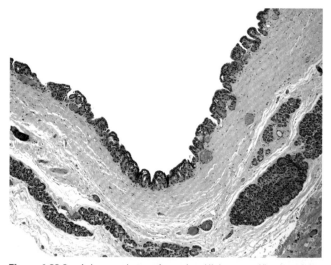

**Figure 1.20.6**    Acinar cystic transformation. Higher magnification of the cyst shown in Figure 1.20.4.

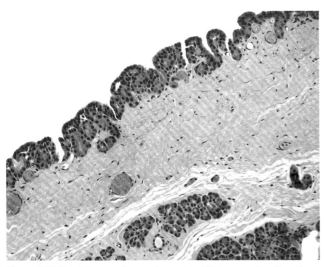

**Figure 1.20.7**   Acinar cystic transformation. Higher magnification of the cyst shown in Figure 1.20.4. Note the one- to two-cell thick layer of pyramidal cells with polarized granular cytoplasm and round nuclei with single prominent nucleoli. The cells lining the cyst are indistinguishable from adjacent normal acinar cells.

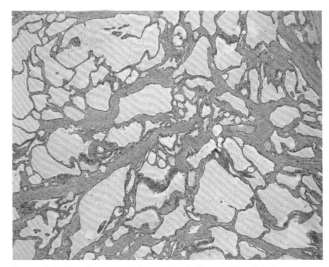

**Figure 1.20.8**   Serous cystadenoma. Note the multiloculated architecture with bands of dense fibrosis.

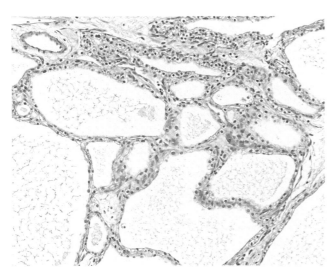

**Figure 1.20.9**   Serous cystadenoma. Higher magnification highlighting optically clear cytoplasm and uniform, centrally placed nuclei.

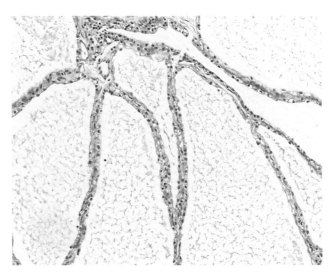

**Figure 1.20.10**   Serous cystadenoma.

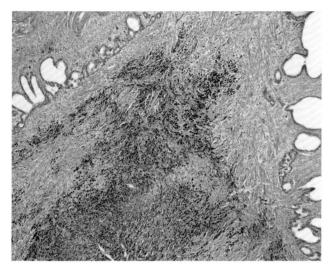

**Figure 1.20.11** Serous cystadenoma. This example shows degenerative changes with fibrosis, hemorrhage, and extensive accumulation of hemosiderin-laden microphages following a fine needle aspiration. Residual microcysts are present at the periphery.

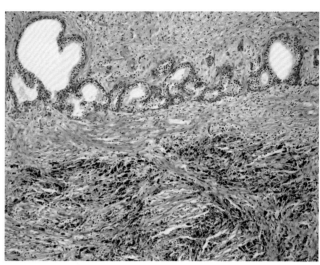

**Figure 1.20.12** Serous cystadenoma. Higher magnification of cyst with degenerative changes shown in Figure 1.20.11.

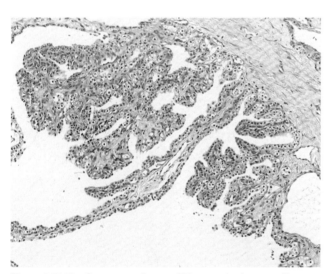

**Figure 1.20.13** Serous cystadenoma. This example shows papillary projections into the lumen.

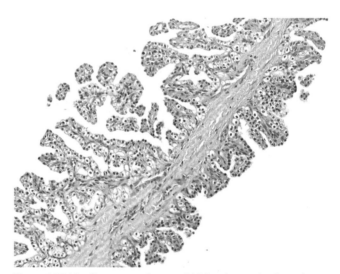

**Figure 1.20.14** Serous cystadenoma. Additional example of complex papillae from the case shown in Figure 1.20.13.

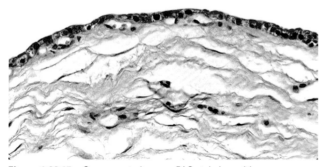

**Figure 1.20.15** Serous cystadenoma. PAS stain is positive.

| | Acinar Cell Carcinoma | Well-Differentiated Pancreatic Neuroendocrine Tumor (PanNET) |
|---|---|---|
| Age | Mean age ~58 y (range 9–89) | Most between 40 and 65 y of age, with a mean age of 58 y |
| Location | Throughout the gland | Throughout the gland |
| Symptoms | Nonspecific. Abdominal pain, nausea, and vomiting | Usually nonspecific, including abdominal pain and nausea |
| Signs | Weight loss. 15% have a syndrome of lipase hypersecretion with fat necrosis, arthralgias and eosinophilia | Solid mass on imaging with enhancement. May be associated with functional syndrome due to secretion of endocrine hormones (insulinoma, somatostatinoma, etc.) |
| Etiology | A minority have deleterious germline variants in cancer predisposition genes including *BRCA2* | Can be seen in patients with von Hippel-Lindau (VHL) syndrome and multiple endocrine neoplasia (MEN) syndrome |
| Histology | 1. Cellular low-power appearance with little stroma *(Fig. 1.21.1)*<br>2. Form acini, or have a sheet-like pattern of growth *(Figs. 1.21.1-1.21.6)*. Occasionally papillary growth *(Fig. 1.21.6)*<br>3. Pyramidal to polygonal cells<br>4. Abundant, often granular cytoplasm<br>5. Polarized neoplastic cells with basally oriented nuclei with single prominent nucleoli *(Figs. 1.21.1-1.21.7)* | 1. Cellular low-power appearance, can have hyalinized vessels or amyloid in stroma *(Figs. 1.21.8-1.21.10)*<br>2. Neoplastic cells form nests and cords. Cells are separated by thin-walled vessels *(Figs. 1.21.8-1.21.12)*<br>3. Rounded or polygonal cells<br>4. Amphophilic cytoplasm *(Fig. 1.21.11)*<br>5. Uniform nuclei with "salt and pepper" chromatin *(Fig. 1.21.11)*. Can see oncocytic differentiation with granular cytoplasm and prominent nucleoli *(Figs. 1.21.12, 1.21.14, and 1.21.15)* |
| Special studies | • Immunolabel with antibodies to trypsin, chymotrypsin, and Bcl10 (carboxyl ester hydrolase) *(Fig. 1.21.14)*<br>• Focal immunolabeling with neuroendocrine markers is common<br>• Immunolabel with antibodies to cytokeratins 8 and 18<br>• Somatic *RAF* gene fusions, among others. Many somatic mutations are therapeutically targetable | • Negative immunolabeling for markers of acinar differentiation *(Fig. 1.21.17)*<br>• Immunolabel with antibodies to synaptophysin and chromogranin *(Figs. 1.21.13 and 1.21.16)*<br>• Immunolabel with antibodies to cytokeratins 8 and 18<br>• Somatic alterations in *DAXX, ATRX, MEN1*, and mTOR pathway genes |
| Treatment | Surgical resection followed by systemic therapy | Surgical resection when possible |
| Prognosis | Fully malignant, with 70% 5-y survival after surgical resection | Malignant. Prognosis depends on grade (proliferation rate) and stage |

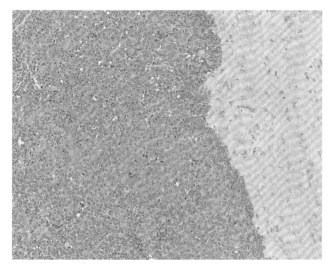

**Figure 1.21.1**    Acinar cell carcinoma. Note the sheet-like growth with scattered acinar formation. Prominent nucleoli are visible even at relatively low magnification.

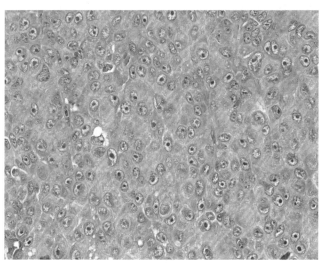

**Figure 1.21.2**    Acinar cell carcinoma. Higher power magnification highlighting granular cytoplasm and single, prominent nucleoli.

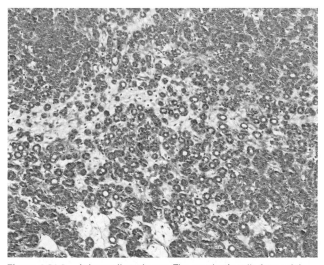

**Figure 1.21.3**    Acinar cell carcinoma. The neoplastic cells form acini. (See chymotrypsin immunostain in Figure 1.21.4.)

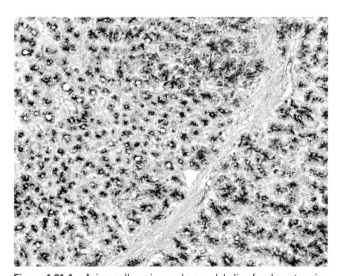

**Figure 1.21.4**    Acinar cell carcinoma. Immunolabeling for chymotrypsin is positive.

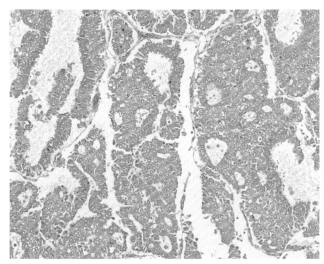

**Figure 1.21.5**    Acinar cell carcinoma.

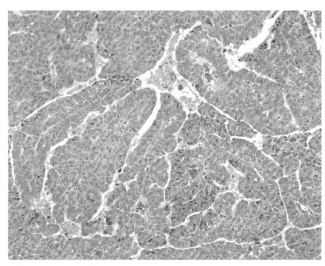

**Figure 1.21.6**    Acinar cell carcinoma. This example has both solid and papillary architecture.

**1.21** Acinar Cell Carcinoma vs. Well-Differentiated Pancreatic Neuroendocrine Tumor (PanNET)    **73**

**1 PANCREAS**

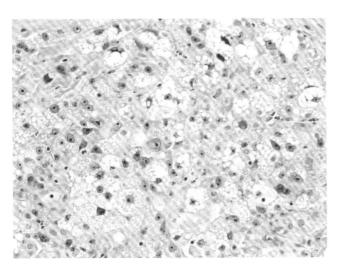

**Figure 1.21.7** Acinar cell carcinoma. This example has lipomatous differentiation. Note prominent single nucleoli.

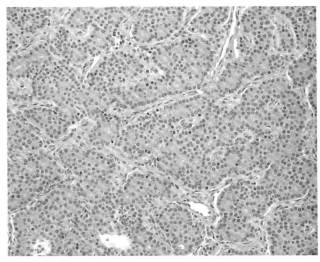

**Figure 1.21.8** Well-differentiated neuroendocrine tumor. Note the nested architecture and delicate vasculature.

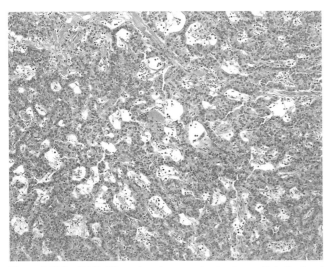

**Figure 1.21.9** Well-differentiated neuroendocrine tumor. Note the focal hyalinized stroma.

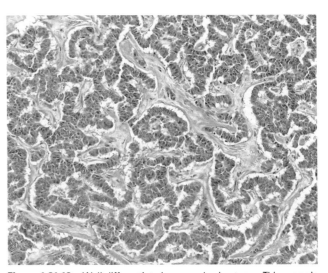

**Figure 1.21.10** Well-differentiated neuroendocrine tumor. This example has a corded/trabecular architecture.

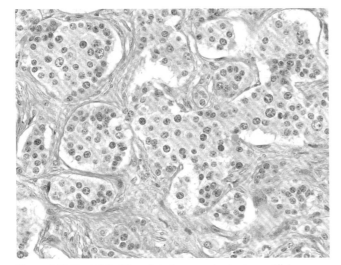

**Figure 1.21.11** Well-differentiated neuroendocrine tumor. Higher power magnification highlighting "salt and pepper" chromatin.

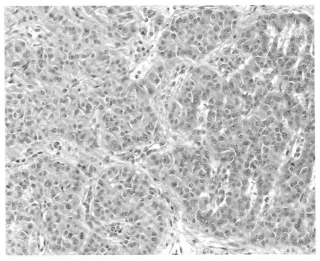

**Figure 1.21.12** Well-differentiated neuroendocrine tumor. This example has oncocytic features with more eosinophilic cytoplasm and nucleoli. The background nuclear chromatin retains a speckled pattern. (See immunolabeling for synaptophysin in Figure 1.21.13.)

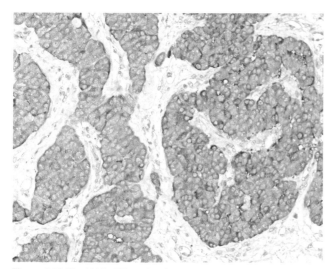

**Figure 1.21.13** Well-differentiated neuroendocrine tumor with oncocytic features. Immunolabeling for synaptophysin is diffusely positive.

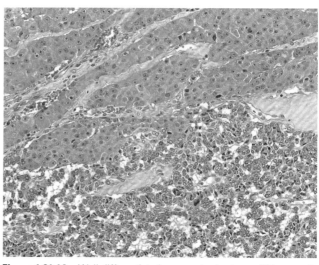

**Figure 1.21.14** Well-differentiated neuroendocrine tumor. This example has classic corded architecture that merges with areas showing well-developed oncocytic differentiation.

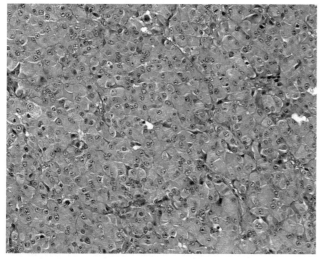

**Figure 1.21.15** Well-differentiated neuroendocrine tumor with oncocytic differentiation. Higher power magnification of the oncocytic component from the neoplasm in Figure 1.21.14. (See immunolabeling for synaptophysin and chymotrypsin in Figures 1.21.16 and 1.21.17.)

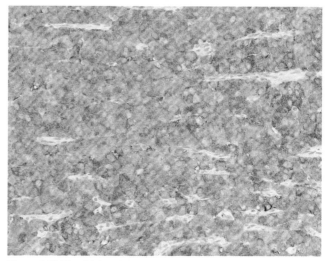

**Figure 1.21.16** Well-differentiated neuroendocrine tumor with oncocytic differentiation. Immunolabeling for synaptophysin is diffusely positive.

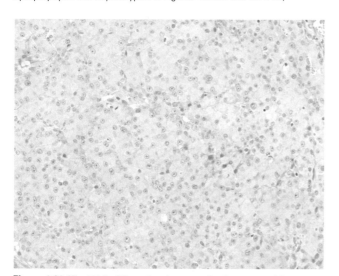

**Figure 1.21.17** Well-differentiated neuroendocrine tumor with oncocytic differentiation. Immunolabeling for chymotrypsin is negative.

| | Acinar Cell Carcinoma With Focal Neuroendocrine Differentiation | Mixed Acinar-Neuroendocrine Carcinoma |
|---|---|---|
| Age | Mean age 58 y (range 9–89) | Mean age 55 y (range 16–89) |
| Location | Throughout the gland | Throughout the gland |
| Symptoms | Nonspecific. Abdominal pain, nausea, and vomiting | Usually nonspecific, including abdominal pain and nausea |
| Signs | Weight loss. 15% have a syndrome of lipase hypersecretion with fat necrosis, arthralgias and eosinophilia | Weight loss |
| Etiology | A minority have deleterious germline variants in cancer predisposition genes including *BRCA2* | Presumably similar to pure acinar cell carcinoma |
| Histology | 1. Cellular low-power appearance with little stroma<br>2. Most are uniform. Acinar formation or sheet-like growth patterns predominate *(Fig. 1.22.4)*. Neuroendocrine differentiation is usually appreciable only with immunolabeling *(Figs. 1.22.5 and 1.22.6)*<br>3. Pyramidal to polygonal cells with abundant, often granular cytoplasm. The neoplastic cells have basally oriented nuclei with single prominent nucleoli *(Fig. 1.22.4)* | 1. Cellular low-power appearance with little stroma<br>2. Most are uniform, but some have two distinct cell populations (one with acinar the other with neuroendocrine differentiation) *(Figs. 1.22.1-1.22.3, 1.22.7-1.22.10)*<br>3. Pyramidal to polygonal cells with abundant, often granular cytoplasm. The neoplastic cells have basally oriented nuclei with single prominent nucleoli. In some instances, but not all, a second component with rounded or polygonal cells with "salt and pepper" chromatin can be appreciated *(Figs. 1.22.1-1.22.3, 1.22.7-1.22.10)* |
| Special studies | • Immunolabel with antibodies to trypsin, chymotrypsin, and Bcl10 (carboxyl ester hydrolase) *(Fig. 1.22.5)*<br>• Focal, <30% of the neoplastic cells immunolabel with antibodies to synaptophysin and chromogranin *(Fig. 1.22.6)*<br>• Immunolabel with antibodies to cytokeratins 8 and 18<br>• Somatic *RAF* gene fusions, among others | • At least 30% of the neoplastic cells immunolabel with antibodies to trypsin, chymotrypsin, and Bcl10 (carboxyl ester hydrolase) *(Figs. 1.22.2 and 1.22.9)*<br>• At least 30% of the neoplastic cells immunolabel with antibodies to synaptophysin and chromogranin *(Figs. 1.22.3 and 1.22.10)*<br>• Immunolabel with antibodies to cytokeratins 8 and 18<br>• Somatic mutations similar in profile to acinar cell carcinomas |
| Treatment | Surgical resection followed by systemic therapy | Surgical resection followed by systemic therapy |
| Prognosis | Fully malignant, with 70% 5-y survival after surgical resection | Fully malignant, similar to pure acinar cell carcinomas. These likely should be considered a subtype of acinar cell carcinomas due to their similar clinical and genetic profiles |

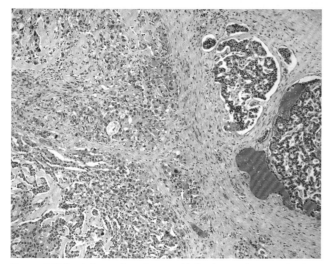

**Figure 1.22.1** Acinar cell carcinoma with focal area of neuroendocrine differentiation. An area at the right of the field has a distinct trabecular architecture and "salt and pepper" nuclear chromatin while the rest of the neoplasm has polygonal cells with granular eosinophilic cytoplasm and prominent nucleoli. The area with neuroendocrine morphology comprised <30% of the tumor. See immunolabeling for Bcl10 and synaptophysin in Figures 1.22.2 and 1.22.3.

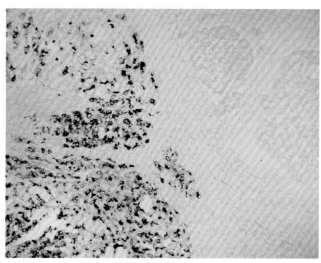

**Figure 1.22.2** Acinar cell carcinoma with focal area of neuroendocrine differentiation. Bcl10 immunolabeling of the case shown in Figure 1.22.1. Note that the area with neuroendocrine morphology does not label for Bcl10.

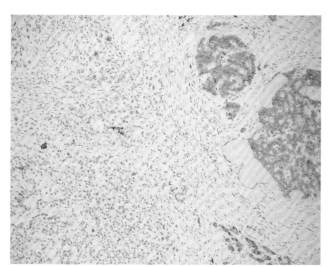

**Figure 1.22.3** Acinar cell carcinoma with focal area of neuroendocrine differentiation. Synaptophysin labeling in the area with neuroendocrine morphology. Note that the remainder of the tumor is negative. The area with neuroendocrine differentiation comprised <30% of the tumor.

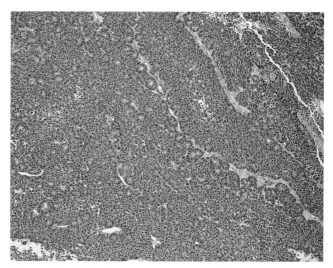

**Figure 1.22.4** Mixed acinar-neuroendocrine carcinoma. This example has a uniform morphology throughout. See immunolabeling for trypsin and chromogranin in Figures 1.22.5 and 1.22.6.

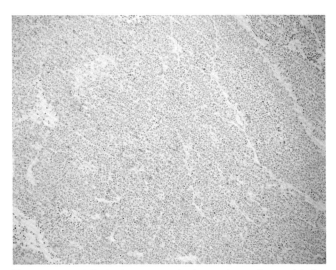

**Figure 1.22.5**    Mixed acinar-neuroendocrine carcinoma. Immunolabeling for trypsin is positive throughout (labels >30% of the neoplastic cells).

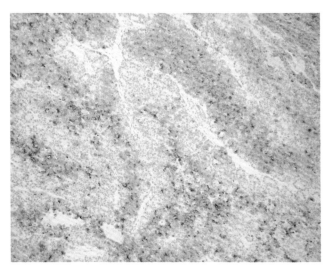

**Figure 1.22.6**    Mixed acinar-neuroendocrine carcinoma. Chromogranin immunolabeling is positive throughout (labels >30% of the neoplastic cells).

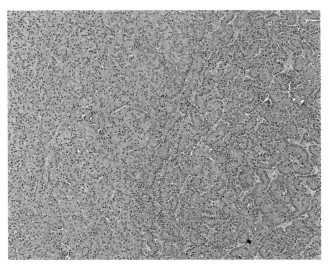

**Figure 1.22.7**    Mixed acinar-neuroendocrine carcinoma. This example shows two distinct morphologies that each comprised greater than 30% of the neoplasm. To the left, the tumor is predominantly sheet-like with polygonal cells with eosinophilic granular cytoplasm. To the right, there is development of more ribbon-like/trabecular architecture. To an extent, prominent nucleoli can be identified throughout, but the background chromatin has a more "salt and pepper" quality. See immunolabeling for chymotrypsin and chromogranin in Figures 1.22.9 and 1.22.10.

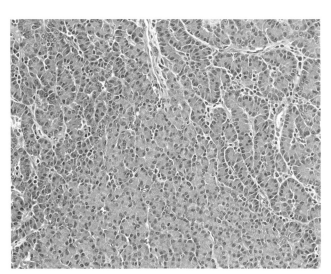

**Figure 1.22.8**    Mixed acinar-neuroendocrine carcinoma. Higher magnification of the neoplasm shown in Figure 1.22.7.

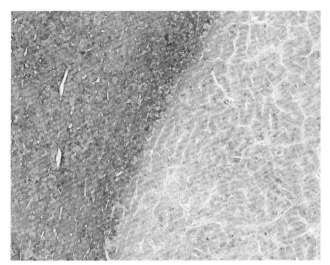

**Figure 1.22.9** Mixed acinar-neuroendocrine carcinoma. Immunolabeling for chymotrypsin is positive throughout but is stronger in the area with more acinar morphology.

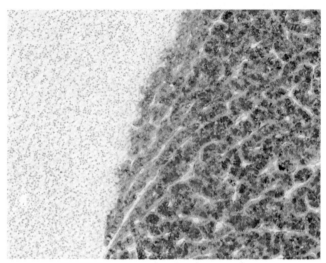

**Figure 1.22.10** Mixed acinar-neuroendocrine carcinoma. Immunolabeling for chromogranin is positive only the area with more neuroendocrine morphology.

|  | Acinar Cell Carcinoma | Pancreatoblastoma |
|---|---|---|
| *Age* | Mean age ~58 y (range 9–89) | Mean age 10 y (bimodal age distribution with two-thirds in children, one-third in adults) |
| *Location* | Throughout the gland | Throughout the gland |
| *Symptoms* | Nonspecific. Abdominal pain, nausea and vomiting | Usually nonspecific, including abdominal pain, diarrhea, and nausea |
| *Signs* | Weight loss. 15% have a syndrome of lipase hypersecretion with fat necrosis, arthralgias and eosinophilia | Weight loss. Palpable abdominal mass |
| *Etiology* | A minority have deleterious germline variants in cancer predisposition genes including *BRCA2*. | Associated with Beckwith-Wiedemann syndrome, case reports in patients with familial adenomatous polyposis |
| *Histology* | 1. Cellular low-power appearance with little stroma<br>2. Acinar formation or sheet-like growth patterns predominate<br>3. Pyramidal to polygonal cells with abundant, often granular cytoplasm. The neoplastic cells have basally oriented nuclei with single prominent nucleoli<br>4. Squamoid nests are absent<br>5. Focal (<30%) neuroendocrine differentiation can be seen | 1. Lobulated, with nests of cellular neoplasm separated by fibrous bands *(Figs. 1.23.5 and 1.23.9)*<br>2. Solid sheets and nests of neoplastic cells. Can see acinar formation in areas of acinar differentiation *(Figs. 1.23.1-1.23.3, 1.23.5, 1.23.7, and 1.23.9)*<br>3. Mixed cell population. Acinar differentiation is invariably present<br>4. Squamoid nests are required for diagnosis. They are composed of discrete circumscribed collections of spindle shaped slightly elongated cells with "hard" eosinophilic cytoplasm. The nuclei are large and often optically clear *(Figs. 1.23.1-1.23.3, 1.23.5, 1.23.7, and 1.23.9)*<br>5. Other components can be present including cells with ductal, endocrine, or mesenchymal differentiation |
| *Special studies* | • Immunolabel with antibodies to trypsin, chymotrypsin, and Bcl10 (carboxyl ester hydrolase)<br>• If present, <30% of the neoplastic cells express synaptophysin and chromogranin<br>• Immunolabel with antibodies to cytokeratins 8 and 18<br>• Normal membranous labeling pattern with antibodies to beta-catenin<br>• Somatic *RAF* gene fusions, among others | • The acinar component immunolabels with antibodies to trypsin, chymotrypsin, and Bcl10 (carboxyl ester hydrolase) *(Fig. 1.23.10)*<br>• Areas of neuroendocrine differentiation immunolabel with antibodies to synaptophysin and chromogranin *(Fig. 1.23.12)*<br>• Immunolabel with antibodies to cytokeratins 8 and 18<br>• The squamoid nests can have an abnormal nuclear pattern of labeling with antibodies to beta-catenin, and because the nuclei of the squamoid nests contain biotin, they can nonspecifically label with a number of different antibodies *(Figs. 1.23.4, 1.23.6, 1.23.8, and 1.23.11)*<br>• Somatic alterations in WNT signaling pathway, most commonly mutations in *CTNNB1* as well as loss of *APC* |

|  | **Acinar Cell Carcinoma** | **Pancreatoblastoma** |
| --- | --- | --- |
| *Treatment* | Surgical resection followed by systemic therapy | Surgical resection followed by systemic therapy |
| *Prognosis* | Fully malignant, with 70% 5-y survival after surgical resection | Fully malignant, prognosis is worse in adults than in children |

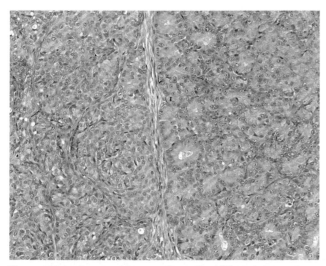

**Figure 1.23.1**    Pancreatoblastoma. Note acinar differentiation on the right with whorled squamoid nests on the left.

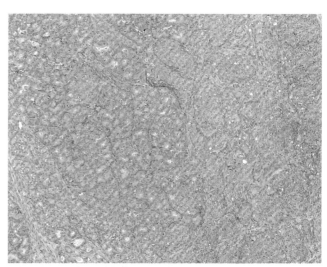

**Figure 1.23.2**    Pancreatoblastoma. Separate area from same neoplasm shown in Figure 1.23.1 with acinar differentiation and whorled squamoid nests.

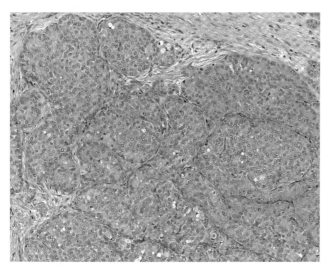

**Figure 1.23.3**    Pancreatoblastoma. Higher magnification image from same neoplasms shown in Figures 1.23.1 and 1.23.2. See beta-catenin immunolabeling in Figure 1.23.4.

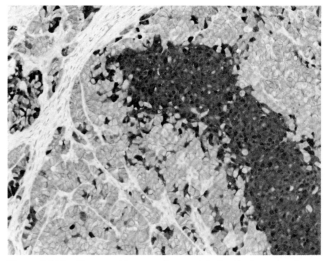

**Figure 1.23.4**    Pancreatoblastoma. Immunolabeling for beta-catenin highlights abnormal nuclear localization in the cells comprising the squamoid nests. Surrounding cells with acinar differentiation show a membranous labeling pattern.

**1.23** Acinar Cell Carcinoma vs. Pancreatoblastoma **81**

PANCREAS 1

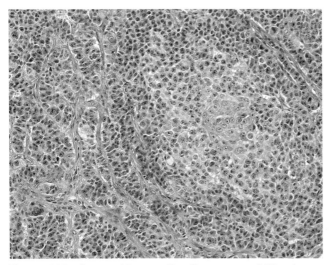

**Figure 1.23.5** Pancreatoblastoma. Note fibrous septae dividing sheet-like cellular growth into lobules and nests with a squamoid nest at the right. See beta-catenin immunolabeling in Figure 1.23.6.

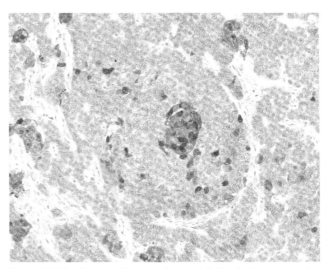

**Figure 1.23.6** Pancreatoblastoma. Immunolabeling for beta-catenin in the same neoplasm shown in Figure 1.23.5 highlights abnormal nuclear localization in the cells comprising the squamoid nests.

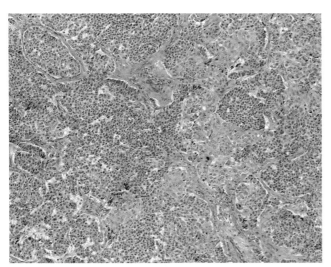

**Figure 1.23.7** Pancreatoblastoma. The morphology in this example is a mix of sheet-like cellular growth and numerous small squamoid nests. See beta-catenin immunolabeling in Figure 1.23.8.

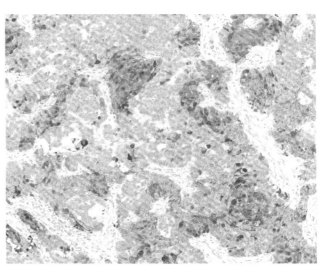

**Figure 1.23.8** Pancreatoblastoma. Immunolabeling for beta-catenin in the same neoplasm shown in Figure 1.23.7 highlights abnormal nuclear localization in the cells comprising the squamoid nests.

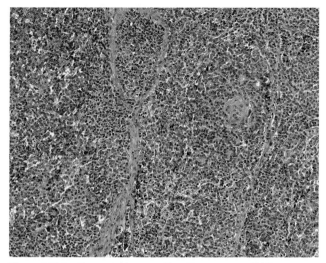

**Figure 1.23.9**    Pancreatoblastoma. Note fibrous septae dividing sheet-like cellular growth into lobules and nests with small squamoid nest at the upper right. See Bcl10, Beta-catenin, and synaptophysin immunolabeling in Figures 1.23.10-1.23.12.

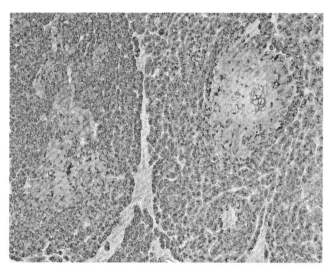

**Figure 1.23.10**    Pancreatoblastoma. Bcl10 immunolabeling in the same neoplasm shown in Figure 1.23.9 highlights extensive acinar differentiation.

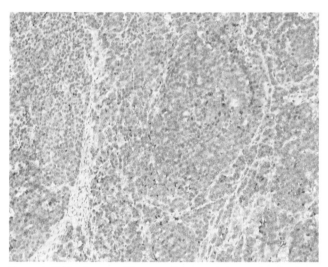

**Figure 1.23.11**    Pancreatoblastoma. Beta-catenin immunolabeling in the same neoplasm shown in Figure 1.23.9 highlights abnormal nuclear localization in the cells comprising the squamoid nests.

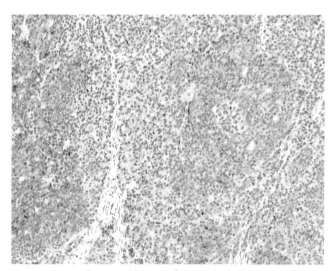

**Figure 1.23.12**    Pancreatoblastoma. Synaptophysin immunolabeling in the same neoplasm shown in Figure 1.23.9 highlights scattered neuroendocrine differentiation.

| | Acinar Cell Carcinoma | Solid-Pseudopapillary Neoplasm |
|---|---|---|
| *Age* | Mean age 58 y (range 9–89) | Mean age of 29 y, 90% female |
| *Location* | Throughout the gland | Tail slightly more often than head |
| *Symptoms* | Nonspecific. Abdominal pain, nausea, and vomiting | Abdominal pain and discomfort, nausea, and vomiting. A third are asymptomatic at diagnosis |
| *Signs* | Weight loss. 15% have a syndrome of lipase hypersecretion with fat necrosis, arthralgias, and eosinophilia | Weight loss |
| *Etiology* | A minority have deleterious germline variants in cancer predisposition genes including *BRCA2* | Unknown |
| *Histology* | 1. Cellular low-power appearance with minimal stroma *(Fig. 1.24.1)*<br>2. Acinar formation or sheet-like growth patterns predominate *(Figs. 1.24.1* and *1.24.2)*<br>3. Pyramidal to polygonal cells with abundant, often granular cytoplasm *(Figs. 1.24.1* and *1.24.2)*<br>4. The neoplastic cells have basally oriented nuclei with single prominent nucleoli *(Figs. 1.24.1* and *1.24.2)*<br>5. Mitoses are common<br>6. Degenerative changes are not common<br>7. Hyaline globules are not common<br>8. May grow within pancreatic ducts | 1. Cellular low-power appearance with minimal stroma *(Figs. 1.24.3, 1.24.14,* and *1.24.16)*<br>2. Poorly cohesive cells, a few of which adhere to delicately branching blood vessels. May see myxoid change in the stroma around vessels *(Figs. 1.24.4-1.24.8)*<br>3. Polygonal cells, some of which can have clear cytoplasm *(Fig. 1.24.13)*<br>4. Round to oval nuclei, some with nuclear grooves. Degenerative-type atypia can be seen, with dark, smudgy nuclei *(Figs. 1.24.7* and *1.24.14)*<br>5. Mitoses are rare<br>6. Degenerative changes including foam cells, cholesterol clefts, hemorrhage and infarction are common *(Figs. 1.24.11* and *1.24.12)*<br>7. Hyaline globules are frequent and often numerous *(Figs. 1.24.8-1.24.10)*<br>8. "Insidious invasion," with minimal stromal reaction in adjacent normal pancreas *(Figs. 1.24.15* and *1.24.16)* |

|  | **Acinar Cell Carcinoma** | **Solid-Pseudopapillary Neoplasm** |
|---|---|---|
| *Special studies* | • Immunolabel with antibodies to trypsin, chymotrypsin and Bcl10 (carboxyl ester hydrolase)<br>• Express cytokeratins 8 and 18<br><br>• May see focal immunolabeling with antibodies to markers of neuroendocrine differentiation<br>• Normal pattern of membranous immunolabeling with antibodies to beta-catenin<br>• Do not express CD10<br>• Do not express CD99<br>• Somatic *RAF* gene fusions, among many others | • No labeling with markers of acinar differentiation<br><br>• Can be negative for cytokeratins or may see focal immunolabeling<br>• May see immunolabeling with antibodies to synaptophysin but no labeling for chromogranin<br>• Abnormal nuclear pattern of immunolabeling with antibodies to beta-catenin *(Fig. 1.24.17)*<br>• Immunolabeling with antibodies to CD10<br>• Immunolabeling in a perinuclear dot-like pattern with antibodies to CD99<br>• Somatic mutations in *CTNNB1* |
| *Treatment* | Surgical resection followed by systemic therapy | Surgical resection |
| *Prognosis* | Fully malignant, with 70% 5-y survival after surgical resection | 5% recur after resection. Very rare metastatic spread. Only 1%–2% die of disease |

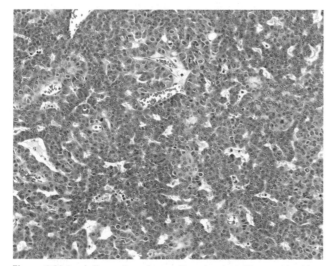

**Figure 1.24.1** Acinar cell carcinoma. Note the sheet-like growth with scattered acinar formation. Single prominent nucleoli are visible even at relatively low magnification.

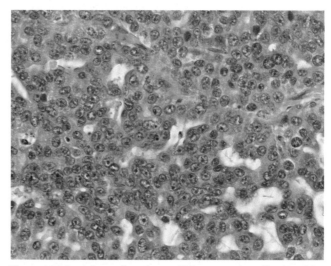

**Figure 1.24.2** Acinar cell carcinoma. Higher power magnification of the same neoplasm shown in Figure 1.24.1 highlighting granular cytoplasm and single, prominent nucleoli.

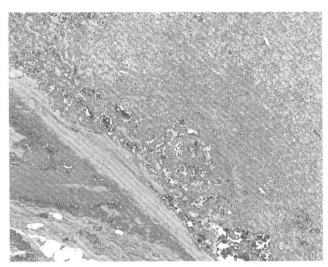

**Figure 1.24.3**   Solid-pseudopapillary neoplasm. Note cellular low-power appearance with minimal stroma and suggestion of poor cohesion.

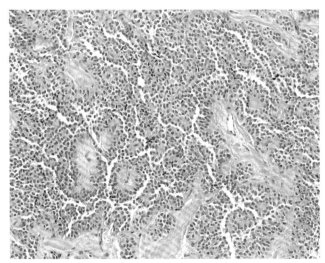

**Figure 1.24.4**   Solid-pseudopapillary neoplasm. Note poorly cohesive cells, a few of which remain adherent to stroma around branching blood vessels forming "pseudo" papillary structures. Focal myxoid change is present around some vessels.

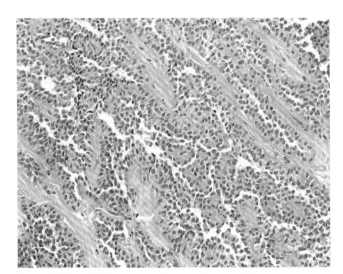

**Figure 1.24.5**   Solid-pseudopapillary neoplasm. Additional view of poorly cohesive cells, a few of which remain adherent to stroma around branching blood vessels forming "pseudo" papillary structures. Focal myxoid change is present around some vessels.

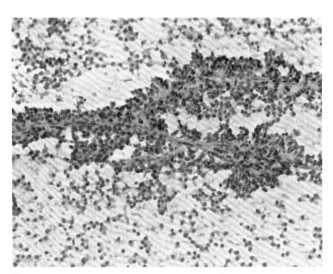

**Figure 1.24.6**   Solid-pseudopapillary neoplasm. Intraoperative smear demonstrating poorly cohesive cells and delicate branching vessels.

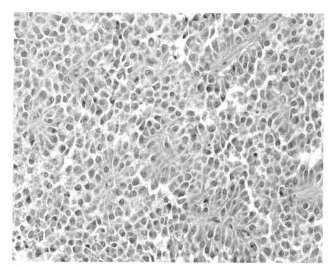

**Figure 1.24.7** Solid-pseudopapillary neoplasm. Higher power magnification of poorly cohesive nature of cells with delicate vasculature.

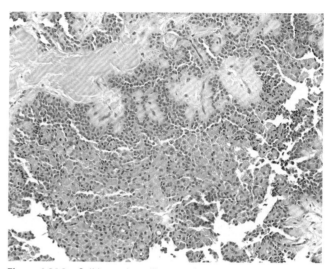

**Figure 1.24.8** Solid-pseudopapillary neoplasm. Note the numerous hyaline globules, and poorly cohesive cells around branching vasculature with associated myxoid stromal change.

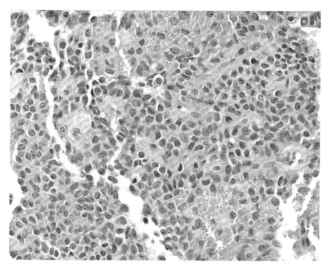

**Figure 1.24.9** Solid-pseudopapillary neoplasm. Higher power magnification of hyaline globules. Also note ovoid cells with nuclear grooves.

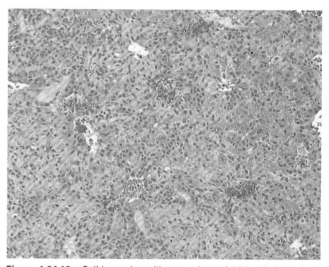

**Figure 1.24.10** Solid-pseudopapillary neoplasm. Additional view with numerous hyaline globules.

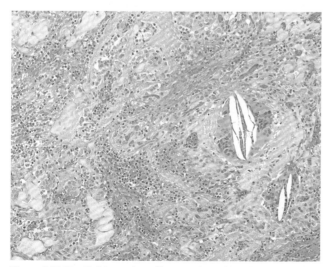

**Figure 1.24.11** Solid-pseudopapillary neoplasm. Note the degenerative changes with cholesterol clefts and multi-nucleated giant cells.

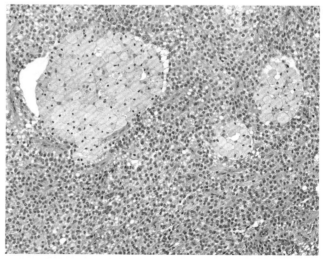

**Figure 1.24.12** Solid-pseudopapillary neoplasm. Note the collection of foamy macrophages. This example also has areas of clear cytoplasm.

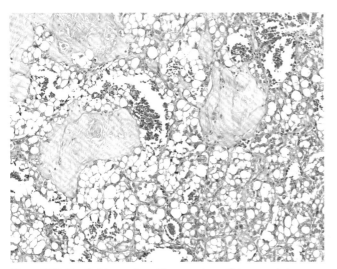

**Figure 1.24.13**    Solid-pseudopapillary neoplasm. This example has prominent clear cell change in the cytoplasm.

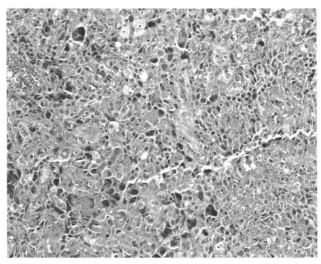

**Figure 1.24.14**    Solid-pseudopapillary neoplasm. Note the smudgy, degenerative-appearing atypia and hyaline globules.

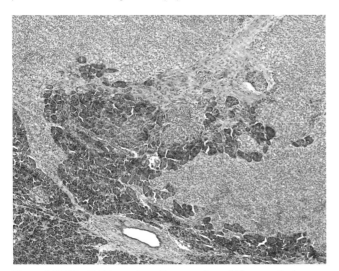

**Figure 1.24.15**    Solid-pseudopapillary neoplasm. This example shows an "insidious" pattern of invasion with neoplastic cells infiltrating around normal pancreatic parenchyma without a stromal reaction.

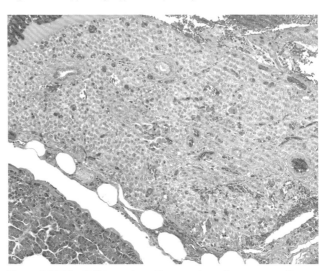

**Figure 1.24.16**    Solid-pseudopapillary neoplasm. See corresponding beta-catenin immunolabeling in Figure 1.24.17.

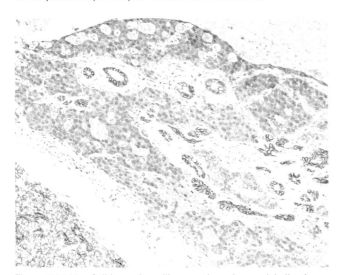

**Figure 1.24.17**    Solid-pseudopapillary neoplasm. Immunolabeling for beta-catenin shows an abnormal pattern of nuclear and cytoplasmic labeling in the neoplastic cells. Note the normal membranous labeling pattern in adjacent pancreatic ducts and acinar tissue.

| | Solid-Pseudopapillary Neoplasm | Well-Differentiated Pancreatic Neuroendocrine Tumor (PanNET) |
|---|---|---|
| Age | Mean age of 29 y, 90% female | Most between 40 and 65 y of age, with a mean age of 58 y |
| Location | Tail slightly more often than head | Throughout the gland |
| Symptoms | Abdominal pain and discomfort, nausea, and vomiting. A third are symptomatic at diagnosis | Usually nonspecific, including abdominal pain and nausea. Functional tumors may be associated with specific constellations of symptoms |
| Signs | Weight loss | Solid mass with peripheral enhancement on CT imaging |
| Etiology | Unknown | Can be seen in patients with von Hippel-Lindau syndrome and multiple endocrine neoplasia, type 1 (MEN1) |
| Histology | 1. Cellular low-power appearance with minimal stroma<br>2. Poorly cohesive cells, a few of which adhere to delicately branching blood vessels. May see myxoid change in the stroma around vessels (Figs. 1.25.5 and 1.25.9)<br>3. Polygonal cells, some of which can have clear cytoplasm (Figs. 1.25.5 and 1.25.16)<br>4. Round to oval nuclei, some with nuclear grooves. Degenerative-type atypia can be seen, with dark, smudgy nuclei<br>5. Mitoses are rare<br>6. Degenerative changes including foam cells, cholesterol clefts, hemorrhage and infarction are common (Fig. 1.25.10)<br>7. Hyaline globules are frequent and often numerous<br>8. "Insidious invasion," with minimal stromal reaction in adjacent normal pancreas | 1. Cellular low-power appearance, can have hyalinized vessels or amyloid in stroma (Fig. 1.25.1)<br>2. Neoplastic cells form cohesive nests and cords. Cells are separated by thin-walled vessels (Figs. 1.25.1, 1.25.2, 1.25.6-1.25.8, and 1.25.15)<br>3. Rounded or polygonal cells with amphophilic cytoplasm. Can see clear cell change (Figs. 1.25.2 and 1.25.15)<br>4. Uniform nuclei with "salt and pepper" chromatin. Degenerative "endocrine-type" atypia with dark, smudgy nuclei may be present (Fig. 1.25.2)<br>5. Mitotic rate defines grade (<2 per 10 HPF, grade 1; 2–20 per 10 HPF, grade 2; >20 per 10 HPF, grade 3)<br>6. Degenerative changes are uncommon<br>7. Hyaline globules can be see but are not characteristic<br>8. Upstream obstructive changes including chronic pancreatitis are common in adjacent pancreas |

| | Solid-Pseudopapillary Neoplasm | Well-Differentiated Pancreatic Neuroendocrine Tumor (PanNET) |
|---|---|---|
| *Special studies* | • May immunolabel with antibodies to synaptophysin but no labeling for chromogranin *(Figs. 1.25.12 and 1.25.13)*<br>• Can be negative for cytokeratins or label focally *(Fig. 1.25.11)*<br>• Abnormal pattern of nuclear immunolabeling with antibodies to beta-catenin *(Fig. 1.25.14)*<br>• Immunolabel with antibodies to CD10<br><br>• Immunolabel in a paranuclear dot-like pattern with antibodies to CD99<br><br>• Somatic mutations in *CTNNB1* | • Diffusely express synaptophysin and chromogranin *(Fig. 1.25.3)*<br><br>• Express cytokeratins 8 and 18<br><br>• Normal pattern of membranous immunolabeling with antibodies to beta-catenin *(Fig. 1.25.4)*<br>• Typically do not label with antibodies to CD10<br>• Immunolabeling with antibodies to CD99 can be variable but does not show a paranuclear-like pattern<br>• Somatic mutations in *DAXX, ATRX, MEN1,* and mTOR pathway genes |
| *Treatment* | Surgical resection | Surgical resection when possible |
| *Prognosis* | 5% recur after resection. Very rare metastatic spread. Only 1%–2% die of disease | Malignant. Prognosis depends on grade (proliferation rate) and stage |

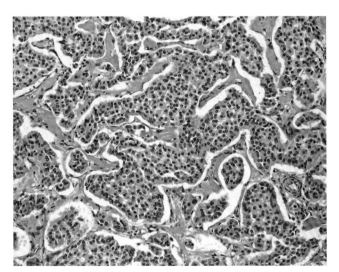

**Figure 1.25.1**    Well-differentiated neuroendocrine tumor. Note the cellular low-power appearance with hyalinized vessels and stroma.

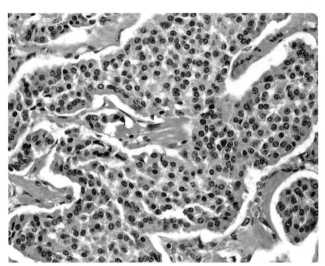

**Figure 1.25.2**    Well-differentiated neuroendocrine tumor. Higher magnification image of neoplasm in Figure 1.25.1. Note uniform nuclei with "salt and pepper" chromatin.

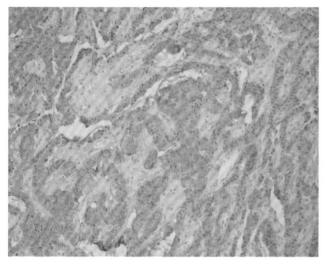

**Figure 1.25.3** Well-differentiated neuroendocrine tumor. Immunolabeling for chromogranin in the same neoplasm shown in Figure 1.25.1.

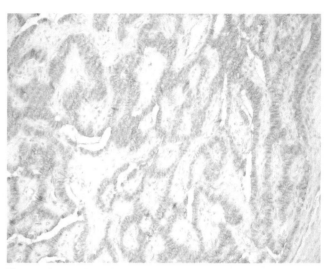

**Figure 1.25.4** Well-differentiated neuroendocrine tumor. Immunolabeling for beta-catenin in the same neoplasm shown in Figure 1.25.1. Note the normal, membranous labeling pattern.

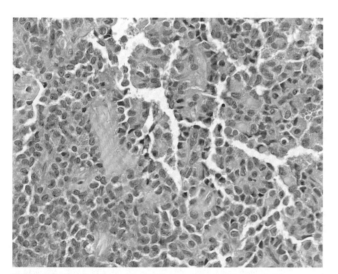

**Figure 1.25.5** Solid-pseudopapillary neoplasm. Note the poorly cohesive cells loosely adherent to blood vessels.

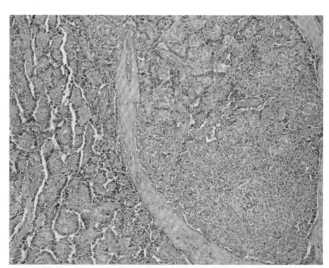

**Figure 1.25.6** Well-differentiated pancreatic neuroendocrine tumor with overlapping morphologic features with solid-pseudopapillary neoplasm. Note the formation of branching pseudopapillae that merge with a more classic nested architecture in the lower right. Nuclear are round with "salt and pepper" chromatin.

1.25 Solid-Pseudopapillary Neoplasm vs. PanNET    91

1    PANCREAS

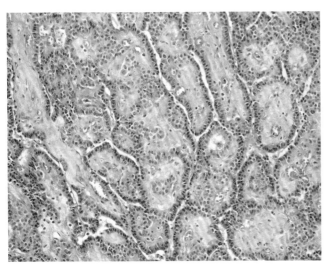

**Figure 1.25.7** Well-differentiated pancreatic neuroendocrine tumor with overlapping morphologic features with solid-pseudopapillary neoplasm. Higher magnification image of neoplasm in Figure 1.25.6.

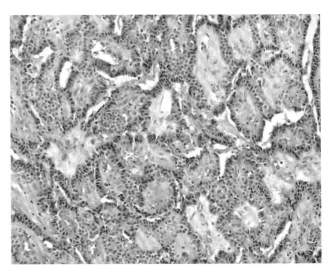

**Figure 1.25.8** Well-differentiated pancreatic neuroendocrine tumor with overlapping morphologic features with solid-pseudopapillary neoplasm. Additional higher magnification image of neoplasm in Figure 1.25.6.

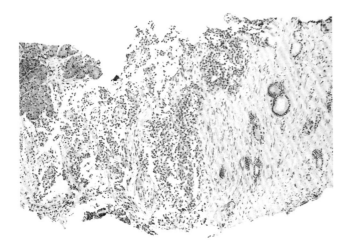

**Figure 1.25.9** Solid-pseudopapillary neoplasm on core biopsy. Note poorly cohesive cells with oval nuclei.

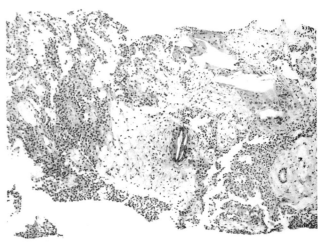

**Figure 1.25.10** Solid-pseudopapillary neoplasm. Note poorly cohesive cells with oval nuclei, degenerative changes, and focal myxoid change in stroma around vessels. See immunolabeling in Figures 1.25.11-1.25.14.

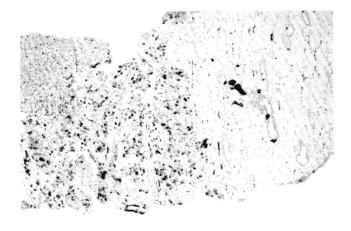

**Figure 1.25.11** Solid-pseudopapillary neoplasm. Immunolabeling for cytokeratin AE1/3 in the neoplasm shown in Figures 1.25.9 and 1.25.10. The labeling is less diffuse than that typically seen in a well-differentiated neuroendocrine tumor.

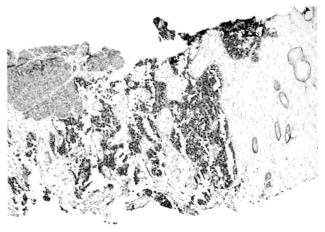

**Figure 1.25.12** Solid-pseudopapillary neoplasm. Immunolabeling for synaptophysin in the neoplasm shown in Figures 1.25.9 and 1.25.10. Labeling with this neuroendocrine marker is commonly seen in solid-pseudopapillary neoplasm.

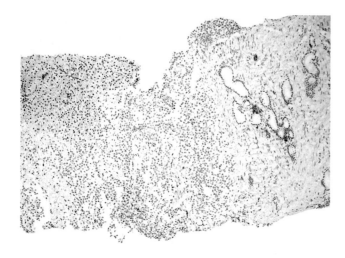

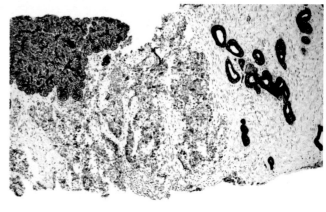

**Figure 1.25.13**   Solid-pseudopapillary neoplasm. The neoplasm, shown in Figures 1.25.9 and 1.25.10, does not immunolabel with antibodies to chromogranin. While synaptophysin labeling is commonly seen in solid-pseudopapillary neoplasms, the neoplastic cells will not label with antibodies for chromogranin. Contrast with labeling for chromogranin in a well-differentiated neuroendocrine tumor in Figure 1.25.3.

**Figure 1.25.14**   Solid-pseudopapillary neoplasm. Immunolabeling for beta-catenin in the neoplasm shown in Figures 1.25.9 and 1.25.10. Note the abnormal pattern of nuclear labeling and contrast with the normal membranous pattern seen in the well-differentiated neuroendocrine tumor shown in Figure 1.25.4.

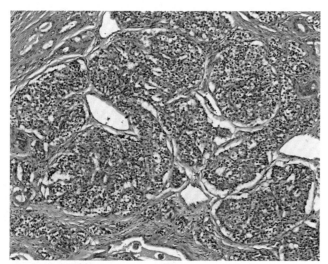

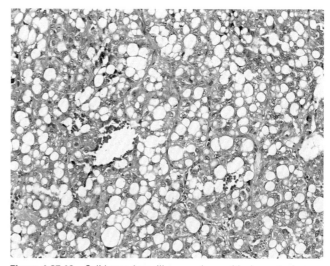

**Figure 1.25.15**   Well-differentiated neuroendocrine tumor showing clear cell change. Note nested pattern with delicate vasculature.

**Figure 1.25.16**   Solid-pseudopapillary neoplasm with clear cytoplasm. Note oval nuclei with grooves.

| | Solid-Pseudopapillary Neoplasm With Necrosis | Pseudocyst |
|---|---|---|
| *Age* | Mean age of 29 y, 90% female | 40s-60s |
| *Location* | Tail slightly more often than head | Extrapancreatic |
| *Symptoms* | Abdominal pain and discomfort, nausea, and vomiting. A third are symptomatic at diagnosis | Abdominal pain, anorexia |
| *Signs* | Weight loss | Abdominal mass after pancreatitis. Tender abdomen on examination |
| *Etiology* | Necrosis may be due to previous fine needle aspiration | Complication of acute or chronic pancreatitis. Often a strong history of alcohol abuse |
| *Histology* | 1. Cysts are intrapancreatic<br>2. Cysts contain necrotic neoplastic cells, which will may be visible as ghosts of cells arranged around blood vessels *(Figs. 1.26.1-1.26.5)*<br>3. A few viable cells may be apparent at the edges of the tumor. Polygonal cells, some of which can have clear cytoplasm, with round to oval nuclei, some with nuclear grooves *(Figs. 1.26.6-1.26.8)*<br>4. Cholesterol clefts and giant cells common<br>5. Hyaline globules | 1. Cysts are usually extrapancreatic<br>2. Cysts contain necrotic debris<br>3. No true epithelial lining. Cyst lined by varied amounts of granulation tissue, mixed acute and chronic inflammation, and foamy macrophages. Associated fibrosis is often present with more cellular areas of stromal change/myofibroblastic proliferation<br>4. Cholesterol clefts and giant cells are less common<br>5. Hyaline globules are not seen |
| *Special studies* | • Immunolabeling often labels even necrotic cells<br>• Abnormal nuclear labeling with antibodies to beta-catenin<br><br>• Immunolabeling with antibodies to CD10<br>• Immunolabeling in a paranuclear dot-like pattern with antibodies to CD99<br>• Cyst fluid may demonstrate somatic mutations in *CTNNB1* | • No neoplastic cells present<br><br>• Normal membranous pattern of immunolabeling with antibodies to beta-catenin<br>• Do not express CD10<br>• Do not express CD99<br><br>• Cyst fluid high in amylase<br>• No somatic mutations detected |
| *Treatment* | Surgical resection | Medical management or drainage |
| *Prognosis* | 5% recur after resection. Only 1%–2% die of disease | ~5% mortality rate |

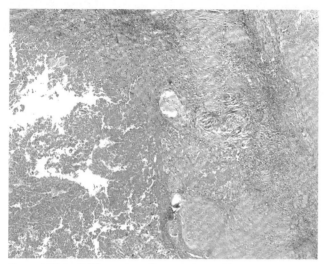

**Figure 1.26.1**    Solid-pseudopapillary neoplasm with necrosis and extensive degenerative changes. Necrotic neoplastic cells are present on the left side of the image.

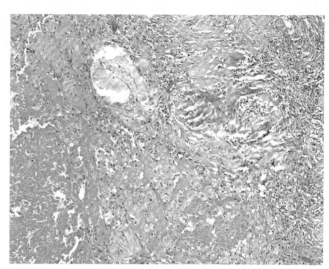

**Figure 1.26.2**    Solid-pseudopapillary neoplasm with necrosis and extensive degenerative changes. Higher power magnification image from same neoplasm shown in Figure 1.26.1.

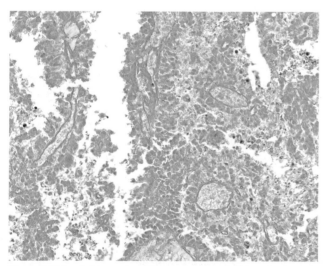

**Figure 1.26.3**    Solid-pseudopapillary neoplasm with necrosis and extensive degenerative changes. Higher power magnification image from same neoplasm shown in Figure 1.26.1. Note necrotic neoplastic cells clinging around small vessels ("pseudo papillae").

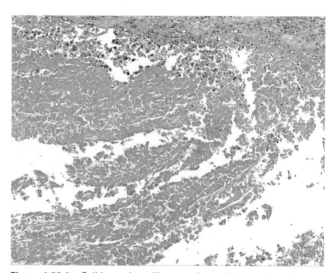

**Figure 1.26.4**    Solid-pseudopapillary neoplasm with necrosis and extensive degenerative changes. Note necrotic pseudo papillary fronds.

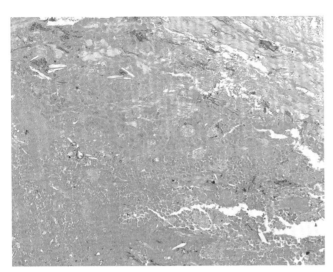

**Figure 1.26.5**    Solid-pseudopapillary neoplasm with necrosis and extensive degenerative changes. Note numerous ghosts of neoplastic cells.

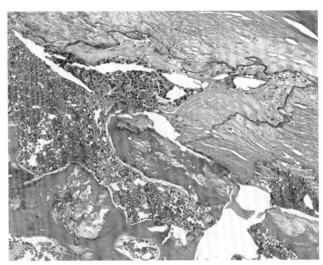

**Figure 1.26.6**    Solid-pseudopapillary neoplasm with extensive degenerative changes including calcification and ossification. Note the residual viable neoplastic cells in the upper half of the field.

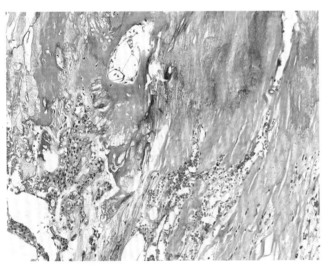

**Figure 1.26.7**    Solid-pseudopapillary neoplasm with extensive degenerative changes including calcification and ossification. Note the residual viable neoplastic cells in the left lower quadrant of the field.

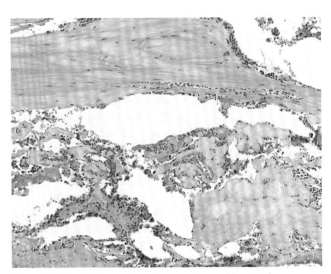

**Figure 1.26.8**    Solid-pseudopapillary neoplasm with extensive degenerative changes and focal residual viable neoplastic cells.

| | Well-Differentiated Pancreatic Neuroendocrine Tumor (PanNET) | Neuroendocrine Carcinoma (NEC) |
|---|---|---|
| Age | Most between 40 and 65 y of age, with a mean age of 58 y | Mean age of 59 y |
| Location | Throughout the gland | Head > tail |
| Symptoms | Usually nonspecific, including abdominal pain and nausea | Epigastric pain, painless jaundice, and nausea |
| Signs | Solid mass with peripheral enhancement on CT imaging | Weight loss and jaundice. Pancreatic mass on imaging |
| Etiology | Can be seen in patients with von Hippel-Lindau syndrome and multiple endocrine neoplasia, type 1 (MEN1) | None known |
| Histology | 1. Circumscribed pattern of growth<br>2. Cellular low-power appearance, can have hyalinized vessels or amyloid in stroma (Fig. 1.27.1)<br>3. Neoplastic cells form nests and cords. Cells are separated by thin-walled vessels (Figs. 1.27.1-1.27.5)<br>4. Rounded or polygonal cells with abundant amphophilic cytoplasm (Figs. 1.27.1-1.27.5)<br>5. Low nuclear to cytoplasmic ratio. Uniform nuclei with "salt and pepper" chromatin. Inconspicuous nucleoli (Figs. 1.27.1-1.27.5)<br>6. Extensive necrosis is uncommon<br>7. Mitotic rate/proliferative index defines grade (<2 per 10 HPF or Ki67 <3%, grade 1; 2–20 per 10 HPF or Ki67 3%–20%, grade 2; >20 per 10 HPF or Ki67 >20%, grade 3), but even grade 3 typically have Ki67 labeling index <55% | 1. Infiltrative growth<br>2. Cellular neoplasm. Can have stromal desmoplasia and geographic necrosis (Figs. 1.27.6-1.27.10)<br>3. Neoplastic cells form sheets or expansile nests with central necrosis, may see rosettes (Figs. 1.27.6-1.27.10)<br>4. Small cell variant has minimal cytoplasm. Large cell variant has more abundant, less granular, cytoplasm (Figs. 1.27.8-1.27.10)<br>5. High nuclear to cytoplasmic ratio. Small cell variant has hyperchromatic nuclei with inconspicuous nucleoli and nuclear molding. Large cell variant has open chromatin, large nests with central necrosis, and peripheral nuclear palisading and can have prominent nucleoli (Figs. 1.27.6-1.27.10)<br>6. Necrosis and apoptotic debris are common (Figs. 1.27.6, 1.27.9, and 1.27.10)<br>7. Very high mitotic rate/proliferative index with Ki67 labeling index typically >55% and often much higher |
| Special studies | • Diffusely immunolabel with antibodies to synaptophysin and chromogranin<br>• Somatic alterations in DAXX, ATRX, MEN1, and mTOR pathway genes | • Diffusely immunolabel with antibodies to synaptophysin and chromogranin<br>• Somatic alterations in TP53, Rb, SMAD4 |
| Treatment | Surgical resection when possible | Surgical resection with adjuvant chemotherapy |
| Prognosis | Malignant. Prognosis depends on grade (proliferation rate) and stage | Highly malignant, with a mean survival only 12 mo |

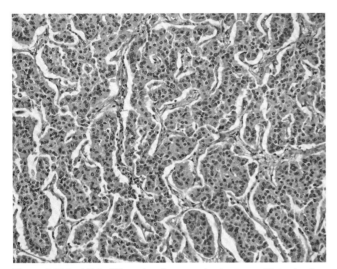

**Figure 1.27.1**   Well-differentiated neuroendocrine tumor. Note classic nested and trabecular morphology.

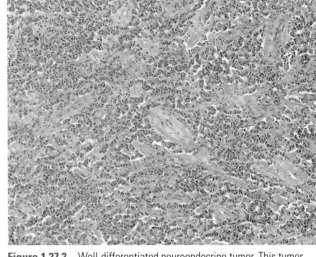

**Figure 1.27.2**   Well-differentiated neuroendocrine tumor. This tumor was WHO Grade 3 with a Ki67 proliferative index >20%. Note the maintenance of a well-differentiated "organoid" architecture.

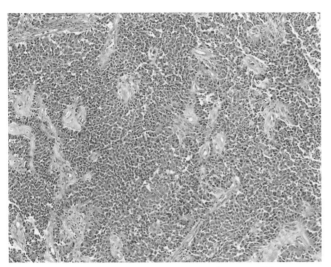

**Figure 1.27.3**   Well-differentiated neuroendocrine tumor. This tumor was WHO Grade 3 with a Ki67 proliferative index >20%. Note that the well-differentiated "organoid" architecture is maintained.

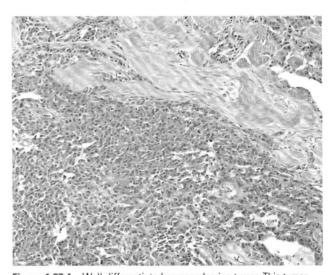

**Figure 1.27.4**   Well-differentiated neuroendocrine tumor. This tumor was WHO Grade 3 with a Ki67 proliferative index >20%. Note that the well-differentiated "organoid" architecture is maintained.

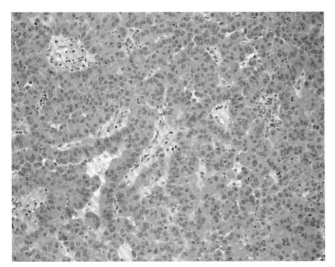

**Figure 1.27.5**   Well-Differentiated neuroendocrine tumor. This tumor was WHO Grade 3 with a Ki67 proliferative index >20%. Note the maintenance of a well-differentiated "organoid" architecture.

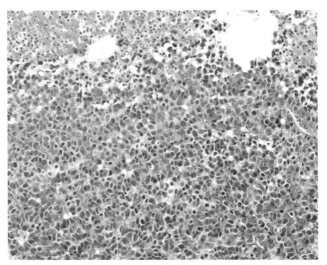

**Figure 1.27.6**   High-grade neuroendocrine carcinoma. Note the sheet like growth, high N:C ratio, nuclear hyperchromasia, and necrosis.

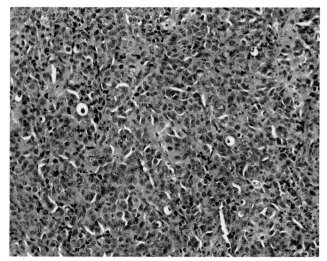

**Figure 1.27.7**    High-grade neuroendocrine carcinoma.

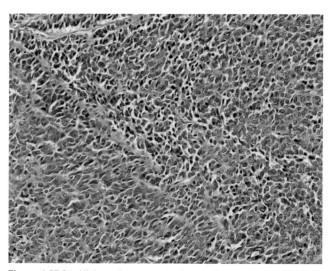

**Figure 1.27.8**    High-grade neuroendocrine carcinoma with small cell features.

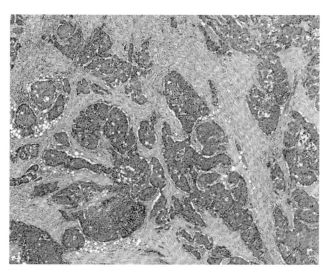

**Figure 1.27.9**    Large cell neuroendocrine carcinoma. Note large nests with peripheral palisading and central necrosis.

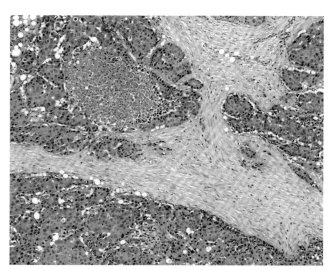

**Figure 1.27.10**    Large cell neuroendocrine carcinoma. Higher magnification image of neoplasm shown in Figure 1.27.9. Note large nests with peripheral palisading and central necrosis.

# ISLET CELL AGGREGATION VS. WELL-DIFFERENTIATED PANCREATIC NEUROENDOCRINE TUMOR (PanNET)

| | Islet Cell Aggregation | Well-Differentiated Pancreatic Neuroendocrine Tumor (PanNET) |
|---|---|---|
| *Age* | Can occur at any age when there is atrophy of the exocrine pancreas | Most between 40 and 65 y of age, with a mean age of 58 y |
| *Location* | Anywhere in the pancreas | Anywhere in the pancreas |
| *Symptoms* | Only those associated with underlying cause of pancreatic atrophy | Usually nonspecific, including abdominal pain and nausea |
| *Signs* | Only those associated with underlying cause of pancreatic atrophy | Solid mass with peripheral enhancement on CT imaging |
| *Etiology* | Atrophy of exocrine pancreas leads to nonneoplastic aggregation of the remaining islets of Langerhans | Can be seen in patients with multiple endocrine neoplasia, Type 1 and von Hippel-Lindau syndrome |
| *Histology* | 1. Small collections of neuroendocrine cells in areas of chronic pancreatitis with acinar drop out *(Figs. 1.28.1-1.28.8)*<br>2. Cells form nests larger than normal islets of Langerhans but the architecture of the islet is maintained *(Figs. 1.28.2 and 1.28.3)*<br>3. The cellular features match those in adjacent normal islets of Langerhans<br>4. The nuclear features match those in adjacent normal islets of Langerhans<br>5. No mitoses | 1. Cellular low-power appearance, can have hyalinized vessels or amyloid in stroma<br>2. Neoplastic cells form nests and cords. Cells are separated by thin-walled vessels<br>3. Rounded or polygonal cells with abundant amphophilic cytoplasm<br>4. Low nuclear to cytoplasmic ratio. "Salt and pepper" chromatin. Inconspicuous nucleoli<br>5. Mitotic rate/proliferative index defines grade (<2 per 10 HPF or Ki67 <3%, grade 1; 2–20 per 10 HPF or Ki67 3%–20%, grade 2; >20 per 10 HPF or Ki67 >20%, grade 3), but even grade 3 typically have Ki67 labeling index <55% |
| *Special studies* | • Diffusely immunolabel with antibodies to synaptophysin and chromogranin *(Fig. 1.28.9)*<br>• Immunolabeling with antibodies to hormonal markers (insulin, glucagon and somatostatin) reveals an admixture of each cell type | • Diffusely immunolabel with antibodies to synaptophysin and chromogranin<br>• Immunolabeling with antibodies to hormonal markers (insulin, glucagon, somatostatin, etc.) may show diffuse labeling with only one marker |
| *Treatment* | None needed | Surgical resection when possible |
| *Prognosis* | Nonneoplastic and completely benign | Malignant. Prognosis depends on grade (proliferation rate) and stage |

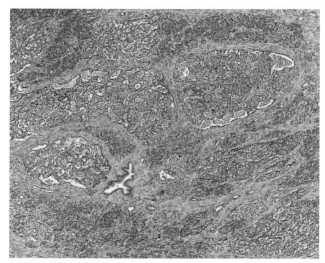

**Figure 1.28.1**    Islet cell aggregation. Background fibrosis and early parenchymal atrophy associated with chronic pancreatitis.

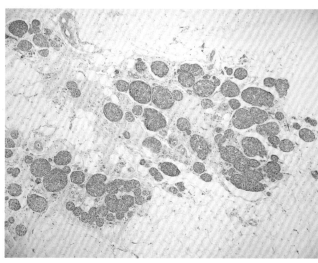

**Figure 1.28.2**    Islet cell aggregation. Note lobulated architecture. Although the islets are larger, their morphologic features are otherwise similar to those of normal islet of Langerhans.

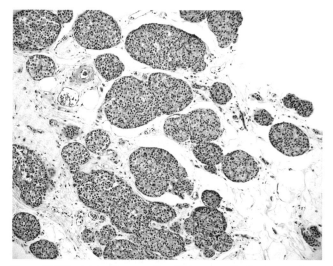

**Figure 1.28.3**    Islet cell aggregation. Higher magnification image of example shown in Figure 1.28.2.

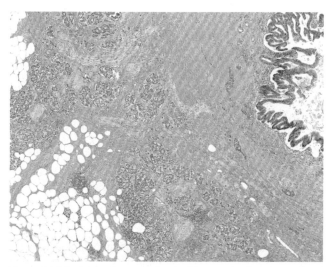

**Figure 1.28.4**    Islet cell aggregation. In this example, there is atrophy of pancreas due to obstructive changes from adjacent intraductal papillary mucinous neoplasm (IPMN) (right side of field).

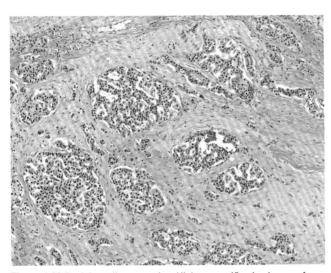

**Figure 1.28.5**   Islet cell aggregation. Higher magnification image of Figure 1.28.4.

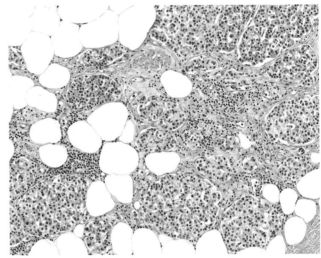

**Figure 1.28.6**   Islet cell aggregation. Additional field from same example shown in Figures 1.28.4 and 1.28.5.

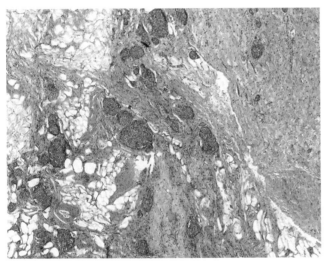

**Figure 1.28.7**   Islet cell aggregation. In this example, there are large rounded collections of islet cells with associated scar suggestive of prior damage and atrophy of pancreatic parenchyma.

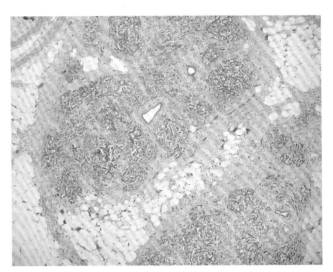

**Figure 1.28.8**   Islet cell aggregation. In this example, the morphology shows a more reticulated/trabecular pattern. See synaptophysin immunolabeling in Figure 1.28.8.

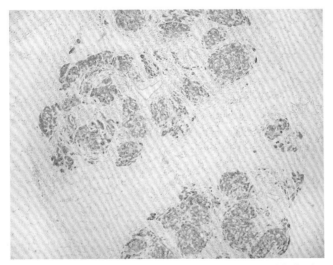

**Figure 1.28.9**   Islet cell aggregation. Synaptophysin immunolabeling in the example shown in Figure 1.28.8.

| | Well-Differentiated Pancreatic Neuroendocrine Tumor (PanNET) With Entrapped Nonneoplastic Ducts | Mixed Neuroendocrine-Ductal Carcinoma |
|---|---|---|
| *Age* | Most between 40 and 65 y of age, with a mean age of 58 y | Mean age of 68 y |
| *Location* | Throughout the gland | Head > tail |
| *Symptoms* | Usually nonspecific, including abdominal pain and nausea | Epigastric pain, painless jaundice, and nausea |
| *Signs* | Solid mass with peripheral enhancement on CT imaging | Weight loss and jaundice |
| *Etiology* | Can be seen in patients with multiple endocrine neoplasia type 1 (MEN1), von Hippel-Lindau syndrome | None known |
| *Histology* | 1. Circumscribed growth pattern<br>2. Cellular low-power appearance, can have hyalinized vessels or amyloid in stroma<br>3. Neoplastic neuroendocrine cells form nests and cords. Cells are separated by thin-walled vessels<br>4. The entrapped ducts may be isolated or in groups retaining a lobulated architecture *(Figs. 1.29.1-1.29.5)*<br>5. Neoplastic neuroendocrine cells are rounded or polygonal cells with abundant amphophilic cytoplasm<br>6. The cytology of the entrapped nonneoplastic ductal cells appears identical to that of epithelial cells in adjacent nonneoplastic ducts *(Figs. 1.29.1-1.29.5)*<br>7. Neoplastic neuroendocrine cells have a low nuclear to cytoplasmic ratio, "salt and pepper" chromatin, and inconspicuous nucleoli<br>8. The entrapped nonneoplastic ductal cells completely lack atypia *(Fig. 1.29.2)*<br>9. Grade of neuroendocrine tumor dependent on mitotic rate/proliferative index<br>10. No mitoses are seen in the entrapped nonneoplastic ductal cells | 1. Infiltrative growth<br>2. Cellular neoplasm. Can have stromal desmoplasia and geographic necrosis<br>3. Neoplastic neuroendocrine component forms sheets or expansile nests with central necrosis. May sometimes show well-differentiated architecture<br>4. Neoplastic ductal component comprised of infiltrative glands, cribriform structures and sometimes individual cells *(Figs. 1.29.6-1.29.11)*<br>5. Small cell variant has minimal cytoplasm. Large cell variant has more abundant, less granular, cytoplasm<br>6. Ductal component varies from normal ductal cells and contains intracellular mucin<br>7. High nuclear to cytoplasmic ratio. Small cell variant has hyperchromatic nuclei with inconspicuous nucleoli, and nuclear molding. Large cell variant has open chromatin, large nests with central necrosis and peripheral nuclear palisading and can have prominent nucleoli<br>8. Ductal component has pleomorphism with nuclear size variation >4:1 and often prominent nucleoli *(Figs. 1.29.6-1.29.9)*<br>9. Mitoses common in ductal component, very high mitotic rate/proliferative index in neuroendocrine component with Ki67 labeling index typically >55% and often much higher |

| | **Well-Differentiated Pancreatic Neuroendocrine Tumor (PanNET) With Entrapped Nonneoplastic Ducts** | **Mixed Neuroendocrine-Ductal Carcinoma** |
|---|---|---|
| *Special studies* | • Neoplastic cells diffusely immunolabel with antibodies for synaptophysin and chromogranin <br>• The entrapped nonneoplastic ducts have intact immunolabeling with antibodies for Smad4 and do not label with antibodies to TP53 <br>• Immunolabeling with antibodies to cytokeratin highlights a lobular, non-random, pattern in the non-neoplastic cells | • Neoplastic neuroendocrine component diffusely immunolabels with antibodies for synaptophysin and chromogranin *(Fig. 1.29.12)* <br>• Neoplastic ductal component has loss of immunolabeling with antibodies to Smad4 in 50%–60% of cases and may show diffuse abnormal immunolabeling with antibodies to TP53. This pattern may also extend to neuroendocrine component *(Fig. 1.29.13)* <br>• Immunolabeling with antibodies to cytokeratin highlights an infiltrative pattern in the neoplastic ductal component |
| *Treatment* | Surgical resection when possible | Surgical resection with adjuvant chemotherapy |
| *Prognosis* | Malignant. Prognosis depends on grade (proliferation rate) and stage | Mean survival only 12 m |

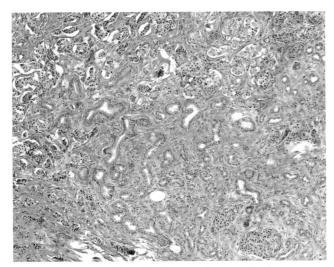

**Figure 1.29.1** Well-differentiated pancreatic neuroendocrine tumor with entrapped ducts. In this example, the tumor extends into an atrophic lobule. Native ducts as well as residual native islets can be seen.

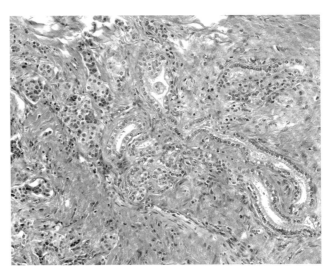

**Figure 1.29.2** Well-differentiated pancreatic neuroendocrine tumor with entrapped ducts. Higher magnification image of tumor shown in Figure 1.29.1. Note the lack of atypia in the trapped ductal cells.

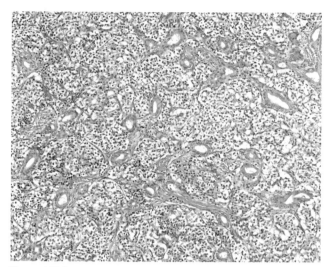

**Figure 1.29.3**   Well-differentiated pancreatic neuroendocrine tumor with entrapped ducts. The nonneoplastic ductal cells are remarkably uniform.

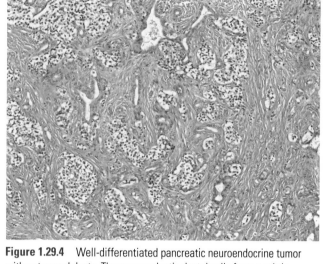

**Figure 1.29.4**   Well-differentiated pancreatic neuroendocrine tumor with entrapped ducts. The nonneoplastic ductal cells form a subtle lobule.

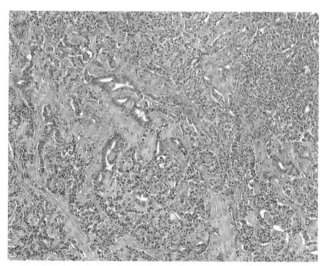

**Figure 1.29.5**   Well-differentiated pancreatic neuroendocrine tumor with entrapped ducts.

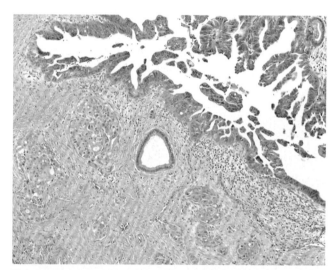

**Figure 1.29.6**   Mixed neuroendocrine-ductal carcinoma. In this example, the adenocarcinoma component is intraductal and the poorly differentiated neuroendocrine carcinoma is in the lower half of the field. Contrast the nuclear features of the single entrapped normal duct to those of the intraductal carcinoma.

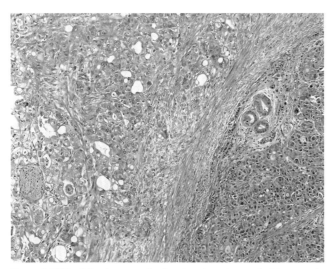

**Figure 1.29.7** Mixed neuroendocrine-ductal carcinoma. In this example a poorly differentiated adenocarcinoma (left) merges with a poorly differentiated neuroendocrine carcinoma (right).

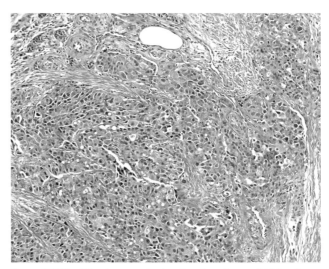

**Figure 1.29.8** Mixed neuroendocrine-ductal carcinoma. Additional image from same neoplasm shown in Figure 1.29.7, predominantly showing the neuroendocrine component.

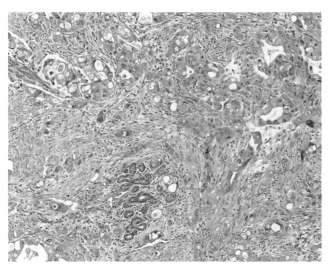

**Figure 1.29.9** Mixed neuroendocrine-ductal carcinoma. In this example, the ductal and neuroendocrine components are intimately mixed. Note the entrapped normal ducts for comparison.

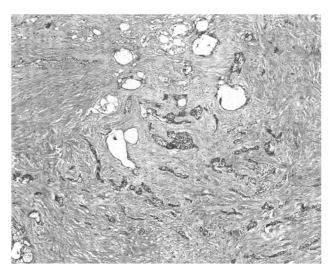

**Figure 1.29.10** Mixed neuroendocrine-ductal carcinoma. In this example, the ductal component has clear cell features and the neuroendocrine component has well-differentiated morphology. See immunolabeling in Figures 1.29.12 and 1.29.13.

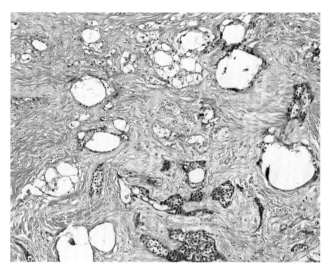

**Figure 1.29.11** Mixed neuroendocrine-ductal carcinoma. Higher magnification image of the neoplasm shown in Figure 1.29.10.

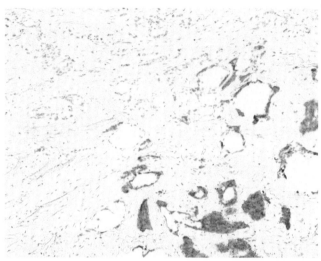

**Figure 1.29.12** Mixed neuroendocrine-ductal carcinoma. Synaptophysin immunolabeling of the same neoplasm shown in Figures 1.29.10 and 1.29.11 is diffuse in neuroendocrine component.

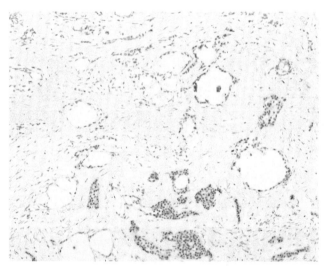

**Figure 1.29.13** Mixed neuroendocrine-ductal carcinoma. Smad4 immunolabeling of the same neoplasm shown in Figures 1.29.10 and 1.29.11 with loss in the ductal component.

| | Well-Differentiated Neuroendocrine Tumor (PanNET) With Clear Cell Change | Metastatic Clear Cell Renal Cell Carcinoma |
|---|---|---|
| *Age* | Most between 40 and 65 y of age, with a mean age of 58 y | Mean age of 65 y |
| *Location* | Throughout the gland | Anywhere in the gland, typically multifocal lesions |
| *Symptoms* | Usually nonspecific, including abdominal pain and nausea | Most are asymptomatic. May have weight loss, abdominal pain, nausea, and vomiting |
| *Signs* | Solid mass with peripheral enhancement on CT imaging | History of renal cell carcinoma. CT scan may reveal an absent kidney from previous resection |
| *Etiology* | Can be seen in patients with von Hippel-Lindau syndrome or multiple endocrine neoplasia Type 1 | Can be seen in patients with von Hippel-Lindau syndrome |
| *Histology* | 1. Neoplastic cells form nests and cords. Cells are separated by thin-walled vessels (*Figs. 1.30.1-1.30.5*)<br>2. Abundant foamy cytoplasm with numerous clear vesicles *Figs. 1.30.1-1.30.5)*<br>3. Uniform nuclei with "salt and pepper" chromatin (*Fig. 1.30.3*) | 1. Polygonal cells with abundant clear to pale, eosinophilic cytoplasm (*Figs. 1.30.7-1.30.9)*<br>2. Sheets or small nests of cells without lumen formation and invested with delicate capillaries. Bleeding and hemosiderin are common (*Figs. 1.30.7-1.30.9)*<br>3. Slightly eccentric nuclei with more pleomorphism. Nucleoli vary with grade and can be prominent (*Figs. 1.30.8* and *1.30.9)* |
| *Special studies* | • Diffusely immunolabel with antibodies for synaptophysin and chromogranin (*Fig. 1.30.6*)<br>• 60%–70% will immunolabel with antibodies to PAX8<br>• Immunolabel with antibodies to cytokeratins 7, 8, and 18 | • Do not immunolabel with antibodies to synaptophysin or chromogranin<br><br>• Immunolabel with antibodies for PAX8<br><br>• Do not express cytokeratin 7 |
| *Treatment* | Surgical resection when possible | Surgical resection if clinically indicated |
| *Prognosis* | Malignant. Prognosis depends on grade (proliferation rate) and stage | Average survival ~5 y after surgical resection |

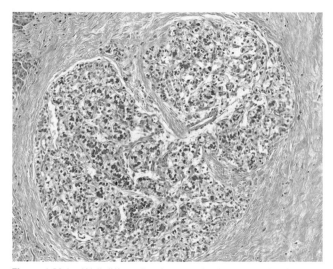

**Figure 1.30.1**    Well-differentiated neuroendocrine tumor with clear cell change. Note the nested growth.

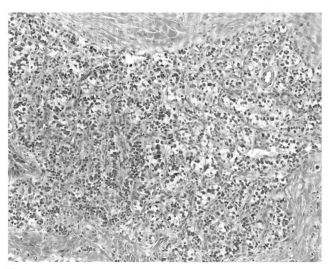

**Figure 1.30.2**    Well-differentiated neuroendocrine tumor with clear cell change. Note the uniform nuclei.

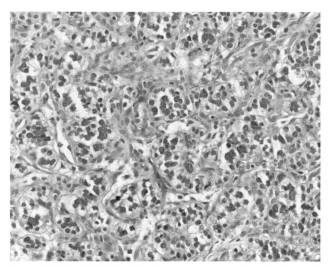

**Figure 1.30.3**    Well-differentiated neuroendocrine tumor with clear cell change. Higher magnification image of neoplasm in Figure 1.30.2. Note the foamy nature of the clear cytoplasm and "salt and pepper" nuclei.

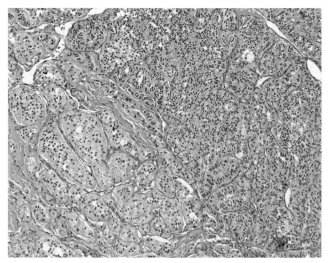

**Figure 1.30.4**    Well-differentiated neuroendocrine tumor. Note focal clear cell changes within the lower left quadrant of the field.

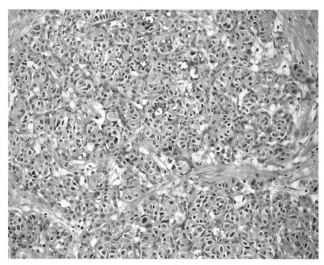

**Figure 1.30.5**    Well-differentiated neuroendocrine tumor with clear cell change. See synaptophysin immunolabeling in Figure 1.30.6.

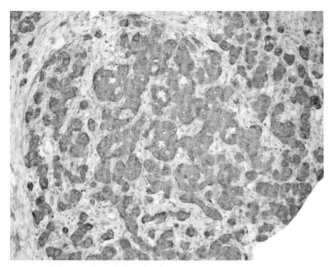

**Figure 1.30.6**    Well-differentiated neuroendocrine tumor with clear cell change. Immunolabeling for synaptophysin in the same neoplasm shown in Figure 1.30.5.

**1.30** Well-Differentiated PanNET With Clear Cell Change vs. Metastatic Clear Cell Renal Cell Carcinoma    **109**

PANCREAS

1  PANCREAS

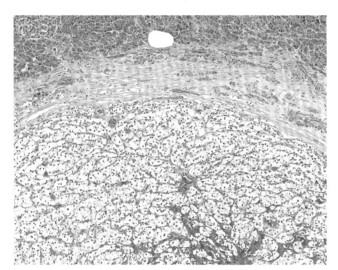

**Figure 1.30.7**    Metastatic clear cell renal cell carcinoma.

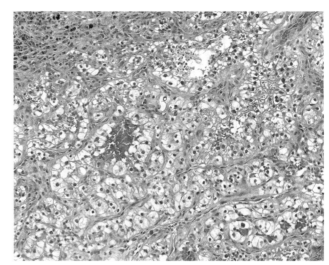

**Figure 1.30.8**    Metastatic clear cell renal cell carcinoma. Note slightly eccentric nuclei with mild pleomorphism and hemorrhage/hemosiderin deposition.

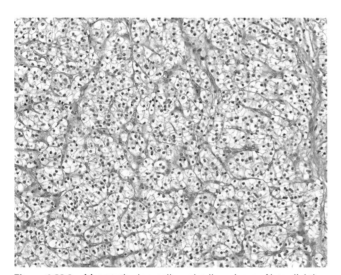

**Figure 1.30.9**    Metastatic clear cell renal cell carcinoma. Note slightly eccentric nuclei with variable nucleoli and sheet-like to nested growth with delicate capillaries.

| | Well-Differentiated Pancreatic Neuroendocrine Tumor (PanNET) | Perivascular Epithelioid Cell Neoplasm (PEComa) |
|---|---|---|
| Age | Most between 40 and 65 y, with a mean age of 58 y | Age range 31–74 y |
| Location | Throughout the gland | Throughout the gland |
| Symptoms | Usually nonspecific, including abdominal pain and nausea | Usually nonspecific, including abdominal pain and nausea |
| Signs | Solid mass with peripheral enhancement on CT imaging | Pancreatic mass on imaging, can be irregular, mixed solid and cystic |
| Etiology | Can be seen in patients with von Hippel-Lindau syndrome and multiple endocrine neoplasia, Type 1 (MEN1) | Can be associated with tuberous sclerosis, but lesions in the pancreas are typically not |
| Histology | 1. Circumscribed growth pattern<br>2. Cellular low-power appearance, can have hyalinized vessels or amyloid in stroma<br>3. Neoplastic cells form nests and cords. Cells are separated by thin-walled vessels<br>4. Rounded or polygonal cells with abundant amphophilic cytoplasm<br>5. Low nuclear to cytoplasmic ratio. "Salt and pepper" chromatin. Inconspicuous nucleoli<br>6. Necrosis is rare<br>7. Grade defined by proliferation rate, but even Grade 3 typically have Ki67 labeling index <55% | 1. Circumscribed growth pattern<br>2. Cellular low-power appearance with scattered thick-walled vessels and rare fat, may see extracellular eosinophilic material and associated calcifications<br>3. Neoplastic cells predominantly form sheets but can also form nests and cords (Figs. 1.31.1-1.31.4)<br>4. Large, epithelioid cells with abundant clear to pink, granular cytoplasm (Figs. 1.31.1-1.31.4)<br>5. Round nuclei with mild pleomorphism, small nucleoli (Figs. 1.31.1-1.31.4)<br>6. No necrosis<br>7. Rare mitoses |
| Special studies | • Diffusely immunolabel with antibodies to synaptophysin and chromogranin<br>• Immunolabel with antibodies to cytokeratin<br>• Do not label with antibodies to HMB45, MelanA, actin, or desmin | • Do not label with antibodies to synaptophysin or chromogranin<br>• Do not label with antibodies to cytokeratin<br>• Immunolabel with antibodies to HMB45, MelanA, actin, and desmin |
| Treatment | Surgical resection when possible | Surgical resection when possible |
| Prognosis | Malignant. Prognosis depends on grade (proliferation rate) and stage | Rare tumor. Prognostic information is limited, but recurrences have been reported. Metastases are rare |

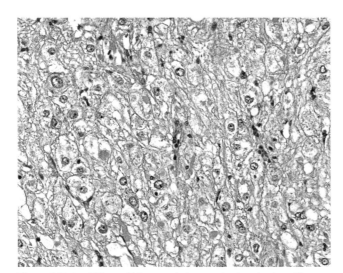

**Figure 1.31.1** PEComa. This example has predominantly sheet-like growth with granular cytoplasm and small nucleoli.

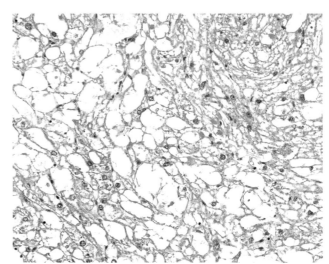

**Figure 1.31.2** PEComa. This additional image from the same neoplasm shown in Figure 1.31.1 shows more cytoplasmic clearing.

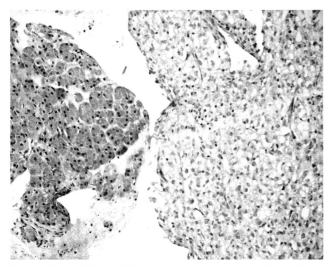

**Figure 1.31.3** PEComa. This example is from a biopsy specimen. Note normal pancreatic parenchyma on the left.

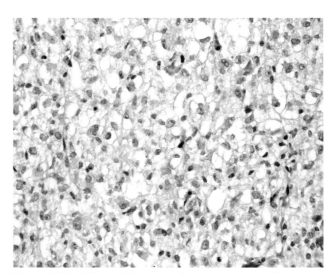

**Figure 1.31.4** PEComa. This example has a mix of eosinophilic and clear cytoplasm with mild nuclear pleomorphism.

|  | Well-Differentiated Pancreatic Neuroendocrine Tumor (PanNET) | Paraganglioma |
|---|---|---|
| *Age* | Most between 40 and 65 y of age, with a mean age of 58 y | Wide age range, median age 39 y |
| *Location* | Intrapancreatic, throughout the gland | Most are peripancreatic, but can occur throughout the gland |
| *Symptoms* | Usually nonspecific, including abdominal pain and nausea | Usually nonspecific, including abdominal pain and nausea |
| *Signs* | Solid, intrapancreatic mass with peripheral enhancement on CT imaging | Solid mass, most commonly peripancreatic |
| *Etiology* | Can be seen in patients with von Hippel-Lindau syndrome and multiple endocrine neoplasia, Type 1 (MEN1) | Can be seen in patients with mutations in genes encoding subunits of the succinate dehydrogenase (SDH) complex |
| *Histology* | 1. Circumscribed growth pattern<br>2. Cellular low-power appearance, can have hyalinized vessels or amyloid in stroma *(Figs. 1.32.1* and *1.32.2)*<br>3. Neoplastic cells form nests and cords. Cells are separated by thin-walled vessels. Can see rosettes or acini *(Figs. 1.32.1-1.32.2)*<br>4. Rounded or polygonal cells with abundant amphophilic cytoplasm *(Figs. 1.32.1* and *1.32.2)*<br>5. Low nuclear to cytoplasmic ratio. Uniform nuclei with "salt and pepper" chromatin. Inconspicuous nucleoli *(Figs. 1.32.1* and *1.32.2)*<br>6. Mitotic rate/proliferative index defines grade (<2 per 10 HPF or Ki67 <3%, grade 1; 2–20 per 10 HPF or Ki67 3%–20%, grade 2; >20 per 10 HPF or Ki67 >20%, grade 3), but even Grade 3 typically have Ki67 labeling index <55% | 1. Circumscribed growth pattern *(Fig. 1.32.3)*<br>2. Cellular low-power appearance with prominent vascular network *(Figs. 1.32.3* and *1.32.4)*<br>3. Classic nested (Zellballen) pattern with variable fibrous banding. May also see trabecular and alveolar patterns. No rosettes or acini *(Figs. 1.32.3-1.32.9)*<br>4. Rounded to oval cells with abundant granular cytoplasm *(Figs. 1.32.3-1.32.9)*<br>5. Low nuclear to cytoplasmic ratio, more prominent nucleoli<br>6. Mitoses are absent to rare. Typically no necrosis |
| *Special studies* | • Immunolabel with antibodies to cytokeratin<br>• Diffusely immunolabel with antibodies to synaptophysin and chromogranin<br>• Do not immunolabel with antibodies to S100<br>• Typically do not label with antibodies to GATA3 | • Do not immunolabel with antibodies to cytokeratin<br>• Diffusely immunolabel with antibodies to synaptophysin and chromogranin *(Fig. 1.32.10)*<br>• Immunolabel with antibodies to S100 and/or SOX10 (sustentacular cells) *(Fig. 1.32.11)*<br>• Immunolabel with antibodies to GATA3 |
| *Treatment* | Surgical resection when possible | Surgical resection when possible |
| *Prognosis* | Malignant. Prognosis depends on grade (proliferation rate) and stage | Rare tumor; malignant behavior is unpredictable and defined only by presence of metastases |

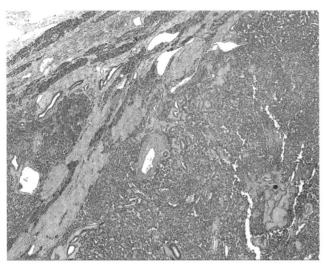

**Figure 1.32.1** Well-differentiated pancreatic neuroendocrine tumor. Note the hyalinized vessels and stroma.

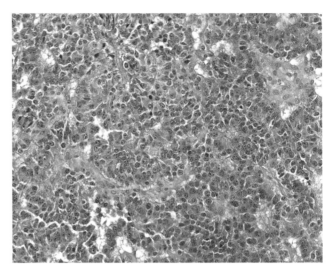

**Figure 1.32.2** Well-differentiated pancreatic neuroendocrine tumor. Higher magnification image of the tumor in Figure 1.32.1.

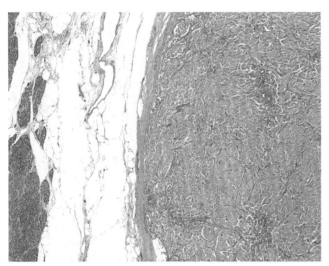

**Figure 1.32.3** Paraganglioma. Note circumscription and peripancreatic location. This example is separated from the pancreas by a plane of fibroadipose tissue.

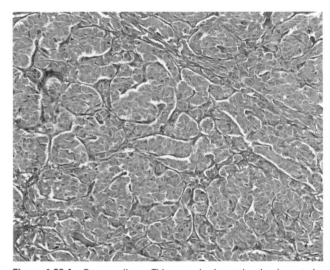

**Figure 1.32.4** Paraganglioma. This example shows the classic nested ("zellballen") architecture with prominent vascular network.

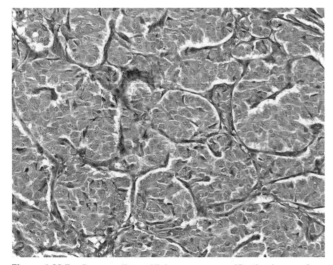

**Figure 1.32.5** Paraganglioma. Higher power magnification image of tumor in Figure 1.32.4.

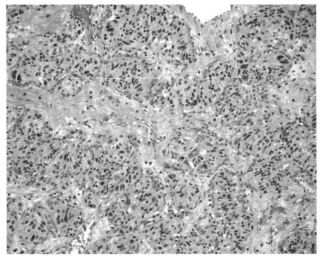

**Figure 1.32.6** Paraganglioma. This example shows a combination of nested and trabecular architecture. Note the oval cells with abundant granular cytoplasm.

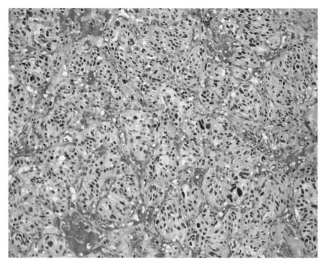

**Figure 1.32.7** Paraganglioma. Higher magnification image of tumor in Figure 1.32.6.

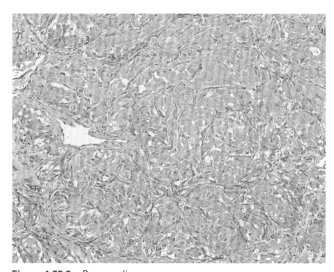

**Figure 1.32.8** Paraganglioma.

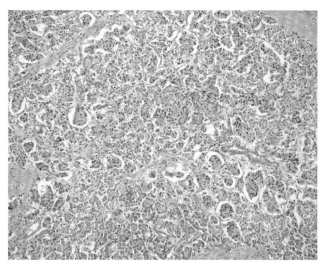

**Figure 1.32.9** Paraganglioma. This example shows a tightly nested architectural pattern.

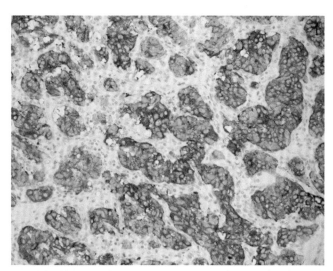

**Figure 1.32.10** Paraganglioma. Diffuse immunolabeling for synaptophysin.

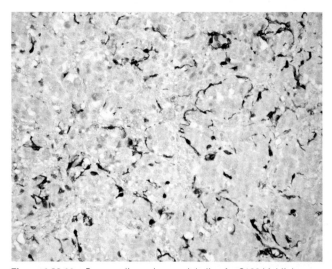

**Figure 1.32.11** Paraganglioma. Immunolabeling for S100 highlights sustentacular cells.

# SUGGESTED READINGS

### Chapters 1.1-1.4

Adsay NV, Bandyopadhyay S, Basturk O, et al. Chronic pancreatitis or pancreatic ductal adenocarcinoma? *Semin Diagn Pathol.* 2004;21(4):268-276.

DeSouza K, Nodit L. Groove pancreatitis: a brief review of a diagnostic challenge. *Arch Pathol Lab Med.* 2015;139:417-421.

Detlefsen S, Klöppel G. IgG4-related disease with emphasis on the biopsy diagnosis of autoimmune pancreatitis and sclerosing cholangitis. *Virchows Arch.* 2018;472(4):545-556.

Hruban RH, Pitman MB, Klimstra DS. *Tumors of the Pancreas. Atlas of Tumor Pathology. Fourth Series, Fascicle.* 6 ed. Washington, DC: American Registry of Pathology and Armed Forces Institute of Pathology; 2007.

Klöppel G, Hruban RH, Longnecker DS, Adler G, Kern SE, Partanen TJ. Ductal adenocarcinoma of the pancreas. In: Bosman FT, Carneiro F, Hruban RH, Theise, eds. *World Health Organization Classification of Tumours*, 5th ed.: Digestive System Tumours. Lyon: IARC Press, 2019:322-332.

Klöppel G, Maillet B. Pathology of acute and chronic pancreatitis. *Pancreas.* 1993;8(6):659-670.

Sharma S, Green KB. The pancreatic duct and its arteriovenous relationship: an underutilized aid in the diagnosis and distinction of pancreatic adenocarcinoma from pancreatic intraepithelial neoplasia. A study of 126 pancreatectomy specimens. *Am J Surg Pathol.* 2004;28(5):613-620.

Shinagare S, Shinagare AB, Deshpande V. Autoimmune pancreatitis: a guide for the histopathologist. *Semin Diagn Pathol.* 2012;29(4):197-204.

Zhang L, Notohara K, Levy MJ, Chari ST, Smyrk TC. IgG4-positive plasma cell infiltration in the diagnosis of autoimmune pancreatitis. *Mod Pathol.* 2007;20(1):23-28.

### Chapters 1.5-1.17

Adsay V, Mino-Kenudson M, Furukawa T, et al. Pathologic evaluation and reporting of intraductal papillary mucinous neoplasms (IPMNs) of the pancreas and other tumoral intraepithelial neoplasms of pancreatobiliary tract: recommendations of Verona consensus meeting. *Ann Surg.* 2016;263(1):162-177.

Basturk O, Adsay V, Askan G, et al. Intraductal tubulopapillary neoplasm of the pancreas: a clinicopathologic and immunohistochemical analysis of 33 cases. *AJSP.* 2017;41:313-325.

Basturk O, Hong SM, Wood LD, et al. A revised classification system and recommendations from the Baltimore consensus meeting for neoplastic precursor lesions in the pancreas. *Am J Surg Pathol.* 2015;39(12):1730-1741.

Basturk O, Tan M, Bhanot U, et al. The oncocytic subtype is genetically distinct from other pancreatic intraductal papillary mucinous neoplasm subtypes. *Mod Pathol.* 2016;29:1058-1069.

Chari ST, Yadav D, Smyrk TC, et al. Study of recurrence after surgical resection of intraductal papillary mucinous neoplasm of the pancreas. *Gastroenterology.* 2002;123(5):1500-1507.

Hruban RH, Adsay NV, Albores-Saavedra J, et al. Pancreatic intraepithelial neoplasia: a new nomenclature and classification system for pancreatic duct lesions. *Am J Surg Pathol.* 2001;25(5):579-586.

Hruban RH, Takaori K, Klimstra DS, et al. An illustrated consensus on the classification of pancreatic intraepithelial neoplasia and intraductal papillary mucinous neoplasms. *Am J Surg Pathol.* 2004;28(8):977-987.

Jang KT, Park SM, Basturk O, et al. Clinicopathologic characteristics of 29 invasive carcinomas arising in 178 pancreatic mucinous cystic neoplasms with ovarian-type stroma. *Am J Surg Pathol.* 2015;39(2):179-187.

Ngamruengphong S, Lennon AM, Analysis of pancreatic cyst fluid. *Surg Pathol Clin.* 2016;9(4):677-684.

Sohn TA, Yeo CJ, Cameron JL, et al. Intraductal papillary mucinous neoplasms of the pancreas: an updated experience. *Ann Surg.* 2004;239(6):788-797.

Springer S, Masica DL, Dal Molin M, et al. A multimodality test to guide the management of patients with a pancreatic cyst. *Sci Transl Med* 2019;11(501):eaav4772. doi: 10.1126/scitranslmed.aav4772

Wilentz RE, Albores-Saavedra J, Hruban RH. Mucinous cystic neoplasms of the pancreas. *Semin Diagn Pathol.* 2000; 17(1):31-42.

Zamboni G, Scarpa A, Bogina G, et al. Mucinous cystic tumors of the pancreas: clinicopathological features, prognosis, and relationship to other mucinous cystic tumors. *Am J Surg Pathol.* 1999;23(4):410-422.

### Chapters 1.18-1.19

Compton CC. Serous cystic tumors of the pancreas. *Semin Diagn Pathol.* 2000;17(1):43-55.

Galanis C, Zamani A, Cameron JL, et al. Resected serous cystic neoplasms of the pancreas: a review of 158 patients with recommendations for treatment. *J Gastrointest Surg* 2007;11(7):820-826.

Hruban RH, Pitman MB, Klimstra DS. *Tumors of the Pancreas. Atlas of Tumor Pathology.* Fourth Series, Fascicle 6 ed. Washington, DC: American Registry of Pathology and Armed Forces Institute of Pathology, 2007.

Panarelli NC, Park KJ, Hruban RH, Klimstra DS. Microcystic serous cystadenoma of the pancreas with subtotal cystic degeneration: another neoplastic mimic of pancreatic pseudocyst. *AJSP.* 2012;36(5):726-731.

### Chapters 1.20-1.24

Abraham SC, Wu TT, Klimstra DS, Finn L, Hruban RH. Distinctive molecular genetic alterations in sporadic and familial adenomatous polyposis-associated pancreatoblastomas: frequent alterations in the APC/beta-catenin pathway and chromosome 11p. *Am J Pathol.* 2001;159:1619-1627.

Hruban RH, Pitman MB, Klimstra DS. *Tumors of the Pancreas. Atlas of Tumor Pathology.* Fourth Series, Fascicle 6 ed. Washington, DC: American Registry of Pathology and Armed Forces Institute of Pathology, 2007.

Klimstra DS, Heffess CS, Oertel JE, Rosai J. Acinar cell carcinoma of the pancreas. A clinicopathologic study of 28 cases. *Am J Surg Pathol.* 1992;16:815-837.

Klimstra DS, Wenig BM, Adair CF, Heffess CS. Pancreatoblastoma. A clinicopathologic study and review of the literature. *Am J Surg Pathol.* 1995;19:1371-1389.

La Rosa S, Adsay V, Albarello L, et al. Clinicopathologic study of 62 acinar cell carcinomas of the pancreas: insights into the morphology and immunophenotype and search for prognostic markers. *Am J Surg Pathol.* 2012;36:1782-1795.

Ordonez NG. Pancreatic acinar cell carcinoma. *Adv Anat Pathol.* 2001;8(3):144-159.

Thompson ED and Wood LD. Pancreatic neoplasms with acinar differentiation: a review of pathologic and molecular features. *Arch Pathol Lab Med.* 2020;144:808-815.

**Chapters 1.25-1.32**

Abraham SC, Klimstra DS, Wilentz RE, et al. Solid-pseudopapillary tumors of the pancreas are genetically distinct from pancreatic ductal adenocarcinomas and almost always harbor beta-catenin mutations. *Am J Pathol.* 2002;160(4):1361-1369.

Akdamar MK, Eltoum I, Eloubeidi MA, Retroperitoneal paraganglioma: EUS appearance and risk associated with EUS-guided FNA. *Gastrointest Endosc.* 2004;60:1018-1021.

Basturk O, Tang LH, Hruban RH, et al. Poorly differentiated neuroendocrine carcinomas of the pancreas: a clinicopathologic analysis of 44 cases. *Am J Surg Pathol.* April 2014;38(4):437-447.

Basturk O, Yang Z, Tang LH, et al. The high grade (WHO G3) pancreatic neuroendocrine tumor category is morphologically and biologically heterogenous and includes both well-differentiated and poorly differentiated neoplasms. *Am J Surg Pathol.* 2015;39(5):683-690.

Heywood G, Smyrk TC, Donohue JH. Primary angiomyolipoma of the pancreas. *Pancreas.* 2004;28:443-445.

Hruban RH, Pitman MB, Klimstra DS. *Tumors of the Pancreas. Atlas of Tumor Pathology.* Fourth Series, Fascicle 6 ed. Washington, DC: American Registry of Pathology and Armed Forces Institute of Pathology, 2007.

Klimstra DS, Perren A, Oberg K, Komminoth P, Bordi C. Pancreatic endocrine tumours: non-functioning tumours and microadenomas. In: DeLellis RA, Lloyd RV, Heitz PU, Eng C, eds. *Pathology and Genetics of Tumours of Endocrine Organs.* Lyon: IARC Press, 2004:201-204.

Klimstra DS, Wenig BM, Heffess CS. Solid-pseudopapillary tumor of the pancreas: a typically cystic carcinoma of low malignant potential. *Semin Diagn Pathol.* 2000;17(1):66-80.

Klöppel G. Pseudocysts and other non-neoplastic cysts of the pancreas. *Semin Diagn Pathol.* 2000;17(1):7-15.

Klöppel G, Klimstra DS, Hruban RH, et al. Pancreatic neuroendocrine tumors: update on the new World Health Organization classification. *AJSP Rev Rep.* 2017;22:233-239.

Manabe T, Miyashita T, Ohshio G, et al. Small carcinoma of the pancreas. Clinical and pathologic evaluation of 17 patients. *Cancer.* 1988;62:135-141.

Sanfey H, Aguilar M, Jones RS. Pseudocysts of the pancreas, a review of 97 cases. *Am Surg.* 1994;60(9):661-668.

Tang LH, Basturk O, Sue JJ, Klimstra DS. A practical approach to the classification of WHO Grade 3 (G3) well-differentiated neuroendocrine tumor (WD-NET) and poorly differentiated neuroendocrine carcinoma (PD-NEC) of the pancreas. *Am J Surg Pathol.* 2016;40(9):1192-1202.

Tang LH, Untch BR, Reidy DL, et al. Well-differentiated neuroendocrine tumors with a morphologically apparent high grade component: a pathway distinct from poorly differentiated neuroendocrine carcinomas. *Clin Cancer Res.* 2016;22(4):1011-1017.

Van Eeden S, de Leng WWJ, Offerhaus GJA, et al. Ductuloinsular tumors of the pancreas: endocrine tumors with entrapped non-neoplastic ductules. *Am J Surg Pathol.* 2004;28:813-820.

# 2

# Ampulla, Extrahepatic Bile Duct, and Gallbladder

| | Chronic Cholecystitis With Reactive Atypia | Well-Differentiated Adenocarcinoma of Gallbladder |
|---|---|---|
| *Age* | Prevalence increases with age | Elderly, mean age 65 y |
| *Location* | Anywhere within the gallbladder | Fundus (60%), body (30%), neck (10%) |
| *Symptoms* | Episodic pain, when calculi are impacted and associated with inflammation, pain lasts >6 h | Two-thirds of the cases are diagnosed incidentally in cholecystectomy specimens, common presentation includes steady abdominal pain and jaundice |
| *Signs* | Ultrasound examination shows stones as movable echogenic objects within the lumen of the gallbladder, cholecystitis characterized by thickened gallbladder wall and pericholecystic fluid | Ultrasound examination shows focal or diffuse mural thickening of the gallbladder and/or an intraluminal mass |
| *Etiology* | Gallstones | Gallstones, known association with primary sclerosing cholangitis, pancreatobiliary maljunction, *Salmonella typhi* infection, Lynch syndrome, and familial adenomatous polyposis |
| *Histology* | 1. The glands are perpendicular to the surface *(Fig. 2.1.1)*<br>2. Luminal tufts present *(Fig. 2.1.2)*<br>3. Luminal bile may be present<br>4. Inflammatory cells frequently present *(Fig. 2.1.3)*<br>5. Although the nuclei may be enlarged, nuclear pleomorphism is absent<br>6. Lymphovascular and perineural invasion are absent | 1. The glands are frequently parallel or oblique to the surface *(Fig. 2.1.4)*<br>2. Open round lumina *(Fig. 2.1.5)*<br>3. Luminal granular debris, luminal bile is absent<br>4. Inflammatory cells usually absent<br>5. Nuclear pleomorphism is present, although it may be mild. Cytologic atypia including prominent cherry-red nucleoli, grooved cell variant, or papillary thyroid carcinoma like nuclei *(Figs. 2.1.6-2.1.8)*<br>6. Lymphovascular and perineural invasion may be present *(Figs. 2.1.9 and 2.1.10)* |
| *Special Studies* | Retained Smad4 immunolabeling | Loss of Smad4 immunolabeling in 50% cases |
| *Treatment* | Surgery | Surgery, chemotherapy |
| *Prognosis* | Excellent | Overall, 5-y survival rate 10%–20% |

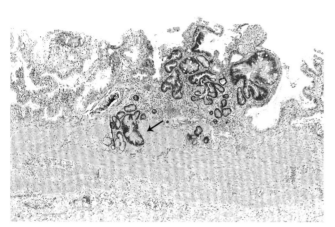

**Figure 2.1.1**    Reactive atypia. Although the deeper aspect of the epithelium is darker, surface maturation is maintained. The glands herniating into the muscle (Rokitansky-Aschoff sinuses, *arrow*) are perpendicular to the surface.

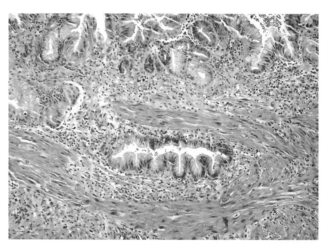

**Figure 2.1.2**    Rokitansky-Aschoff sinuses. These pathologic herniations of the mucosa into or though the muscularis are analogous to intestinal diverticula. Increased luminal pressure causes this herniation of the epithelium and the herniations are commonly associated with the obstruction of biliary outflow often caused by the gallstones. Luminal tufts are present in the reactive glands.

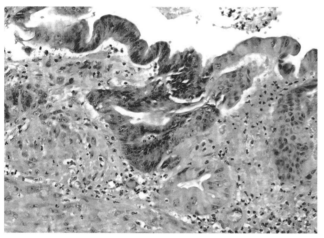

**Figure 2.1.3**    Reactive atypia. Acute inflammatory cells are often present in reactive changes. When hemorrhage is present in the stroma, epithelial atypia should be interpreted with caution. Evenness of nuclear chromatin, lack of marked nuclear enlargement and sharp and smooth chromatin, all support reactive changes.

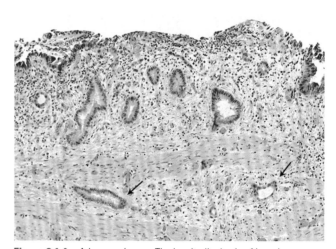

**Figure 2.1.4**    Adenocarcinoma. The longitudinal axis of invasive carcinoma is parallel to the surface (*arrows*). Luminal tufts are absent.

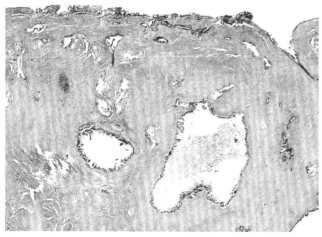

**Figure 2.1.5**    Adenocarcinoma. The glands of invasive carcinoma may have open round lumina with irregular contours. Cellular debris is present in the lumina.

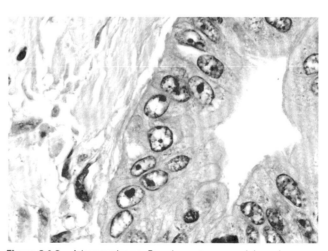

**Figure 2.1.6**    Adenocarcinoma. Round monotonous nuclei may have prominent cherry-red nucleoli.

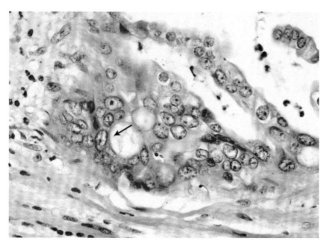

**Figure 2.1.7** Adenocarcinoma, grooved cell variant. Nuclei of the neoplastic cells may have grooves (*arrow*) without nucleoli.

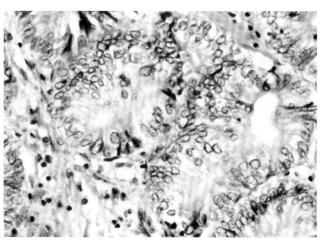

**Figure 2.1.8** Adenocarcinoma, papillary thyroid carcinoma–like variant. Neoplastic glands with overlapping bland nuclei with chromatin clearing similar to papillary thyroid carcinoma.

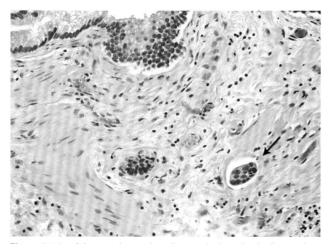

**Figure 2.1.9** Adenocarcinoma. Lymphovascular invasion is diagnostic (*arrow*).

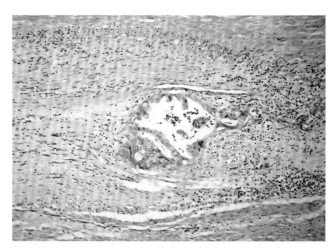

**Figure 2.1.10** Adenocarcinoma. Perineural invasion is virtually diagnostic.

| | Chronic Cholecystitis With Signet Ring Cell Changes | Adenocarcinoma of Gallbladder With Signet Ring Cells |
|---|---|---|
| Age | Reported in the young and elderly | Reported in young men without cholelithiasis |
| Location | Anywhere within the gallbladder | Anywhere within the gallbladder |
| Symptom | Episodic pain, when stone is impacted and associated with inflammation, pain lasts >6 h | Two thirds of the cases are diagnosed incidentally in cholecystectomy specimens. When symptomatic, common presentation includes steady abdominal pain and jaundice |
| Signs | Ultrasound examination shows thickened gallbladder wall and pericholecystic fluid | Ultrasound examination shows focal or diffuse mural thickening of the gallbladder and an intraluminal mass |
| Etiology | Artifact caused by sloughing and disaggregation of the epithelial cells often related to ischemia | Accumulation of mucin in the cytoplasm of malignant epithelial cells |
| Histology | 1. Signet ring cells are confined to the surface of the mucosa or the glandular lumina *(Figs. 2.2.1 and 2.2.2)*<br>2. Admixture with histiocytes and other inflammatory cells with necrotizing changes *(Fig. 2.2.3)*<br>3. Lack of nuclear atypia, nuclear hyperchromasia, prominent nucleoli and mitosis *(Fig. 2.2.4)*<br>4. Positive for mucicarmine | 1. Signet cells infiltrate into the lamina propria *(Fig. 2.2.7)*<br>2. Nuclear atypia *(Fig. 2.2.8)*<br>3. Inflammation is mild<br>4. Positive for mucicarmine |
| Special Studies | • Express cytokeratin *(Fig. 2.2.5)*<br>• Intact E-cadherin expression *(Fig. 2.2.6)*<br>• No *TP53* mutations | • Express cytokeratin<br>• E-cadherin loss<br>• Can have *TP53* mutations |
| Treatment | Surgery | Surgery, chemotherapy |
| Prognosis | Overdiagnosis as signet ring cell adenocarcinoma risks overtreatment; otherwise, excellent prognosis | Highly aggressive malignancy with poor prognosis |

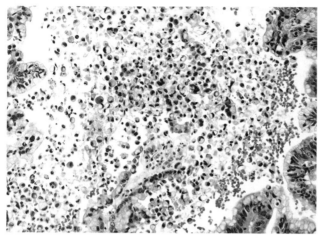

**Figure 2.2.1**  Chronic cholecystitis with signet ring cell changes. Signet ring cells changes are confined to the surface of the mucosa.

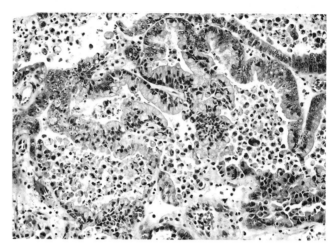

**Figure 2.2.2**  Chronic cholecystitis with signet ring cell changes. Signet ring cell changes are confined to the inside of glandular lumina.

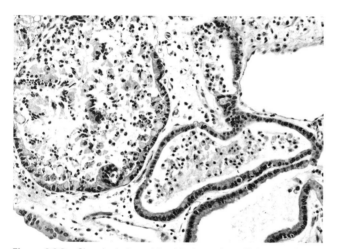

**Figure 2.2.3**  Chronic cholecystitis with signet ring cell changes. Signet ring cell changes are confined to the inside of glandular lumina and admixed with histiocytes and other inflammatory cells.

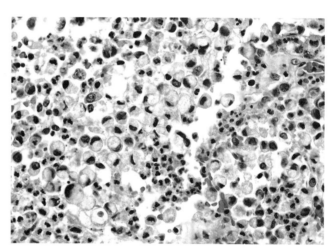

**Figure 2.2.4**  Chronic cholecystitis with signet ring cell changes. Signet ring cell changes lack nuclear atypia, hyperchromasia, and mitosis.

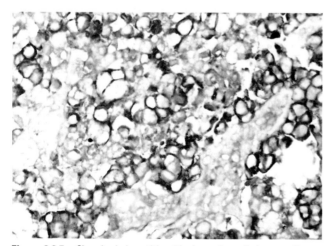

**Figure 2.2.5**  Chronic cholecystitis with signet ring cell changes. Signet ring cell changes immunolabel with antibodies to keratin (AE1/3) and immunolabeling does not help to differentiate signet ring cell changes from carcinoma.

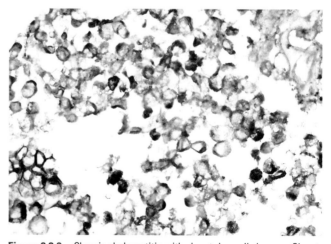

**Figure 2.2.6**  Chronic cholecystitis with signet ring cell changes. Signet ring cell changes express E-cadherin and the intact labeling supports reactive changes.

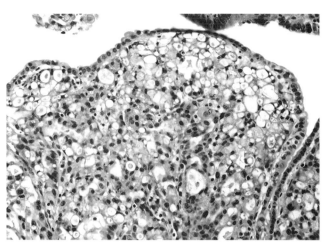

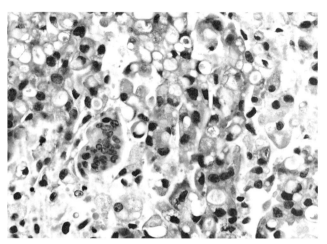

**Figure 2.2.7**   Signet ring cell carcinoma. The neoplastic cells infiltrate into the lamina propria.

**Figure 2.2.8**   Signet ring cell carcinoma. Note the nuclear atypia.

|  | **Chronic Cholecystitis With Reactive Atypia** | **Gallbladder With Dysplasia** |
|---|---|---|
| *Age* | The prevalence increases with age | Early 60s |
| *Location* | Anywhere within the gallbladder | Anywhere within the gallbladder |
| *Symptom* | Episodic pain, when calculi are impacted and associated with inflammation, pain lasts >6 h | Usually an incidental finding in gallbladders removed for other disorders |
| *Signs* | Ultrasound examination shows thickened gallbladder wall and pericholecystic fluid | None |
| *Etiology* | Gallstones | Gallstones, associated with primary sclerosing cholangitis, pancreatobiliary maljunction, porcelain gallbladder, *Salmonella typhi* infection, Lynch syndrome, and familial adenomatous polyposis |
| *Histology* | 1. Complex architecture is absent<br>2. Nuclear enlargement is absent *(Fig. 2.3.1)*<br>3. Hyper and hypochromatic nuclei<br>4. Surface maturation present<br>5. Inflammatory cells present<br>6. Stromal hemorrhage and edema present *(Fig. 2.3.2)*<br>7. Goblet cells are absent<br>8. Mitotic figures may be present, but have a normal morphology *(Fig. 2.3.3)* | 1. Papillary, micropapillary, tufting, cribriform arrangements are present *(Figs. 2.3.3-2.3.5)*<br>2. Nuclear enlargement with very large prominent cherry-red nucleoli<br>3. Hyperchromatic nuclei *(Fig. 2.3.6)*<br>4. Surface maturation absent<br>5. Inflammatory cells are not present<br>6. Stromal hemorrhage and edema are absent<br>7. Goblet cells may be present *(Fig. 2.3.7)*<br>8. Mitotic figures may be present, and may have an abnormal morphology |
| *Special Studies* | • TP53 immunolabeling is negative | • TP53 immunolabeling:<br>  Low grade = negative<br>  High grade = frequently positive |
| *Treatment* | Surgery may be indicated | Incidental finding, no further treatment |
| *Prognosis* | Excellent | Depends on associated disorder |

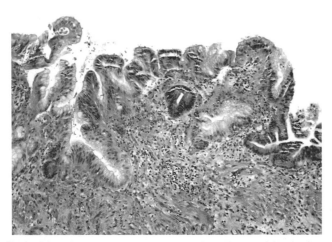

**Figure 2.3.1** Reactive atypia. Although the deeper aspect of the glands is darker, surface maturation is maintained. Chromatin is smooth and even, and there is no nuclear enlargement.

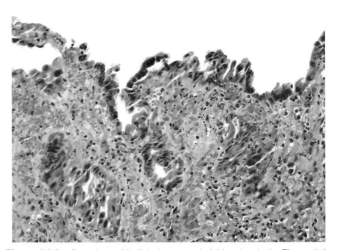

**Figure 2.3.2** Reactive epithelial changes mimicking dysplasia. The nuclei have mild atypia, they are disorganized and relatively hypochromatic. There is hemorrhage and inflammation in the stroma indicating an area of injury.

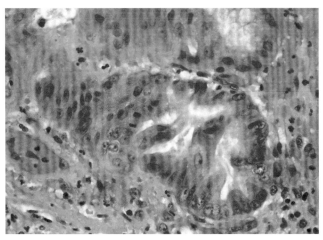

**Figure 2.3.3**   Reactive atypia. Mitotic figures may be present in reactive changes, but have a normal morphology.

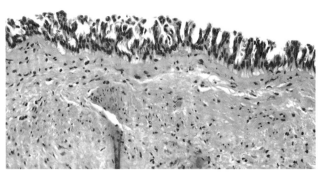

**Figure 2.3.4**   Gallbladder with dysplasia. The architecture is often complex, such as micropapillary in this case.

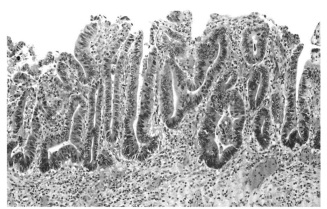

**Figure 2.3.5**   Gallbladder with dysplasia. High-grade dysplasia with a relatively monotonous appearance, but cytologic atypia characterized by a high nucleus to cytoplasm ratio is noted.

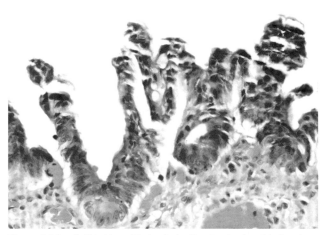

**Figure 2.3.6**   Gallbladder with dysplasia. The dysplastic epithelium is hyperchromatic and has enlarged nuclei. Surface maturation is absent.

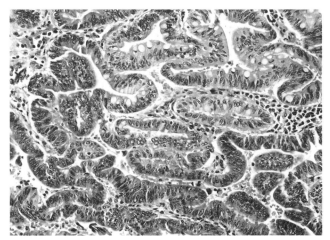

**Figure 2.3.7**   Gallbladder with dysplasia. The epithelium with high-grade dysplasia has intestinal differentiation metaplasia.

| | Pyloric Gland Adenoma (PGA) | Intracholecystic Papillary Neoplasm (ICPN) |
|---|---|---|
| *Age* | 46–76 y of age (mean: 61 y) | 20–94 y of age (mean:61 y) |
| *Location* | Anywhere within the gallbladder | Anywhere within the gallbladder |
| *Sex* | More common in females | Female: male ratio of 2:1 |
| *Symptom* | Often asymptomatic when <2 cm | Right upper quadrant abdominal pain |
| *Signs* | Imaging, including abdominal ultrasound, can detect most cases | Half of the cases are diagnosed as gallbladder cancer radiologically |
| *Etiology* | Unknown. Half of the cases are associated with cholelithiasis. Occasionally associated with Peutz-Jeghers syndrome or familial adenomatous polyposis | Unknown. No association with gallstones |
| *Histology* | 1. Sessile or pedunculated configuration (*Figs. 2.4.1* and *2.4.2*). If the nodule is less than 0.5 cm and arises in a background of pyloric metaplasia in the adjacent mucosa, it should be called polypoid pyloric metaplasia, not PGA (*Fig. 2.4.3*)<br>2. Tightly packed bland-looking pyloric type or Brunner gland-like glands (*Figs. 2.4.4* and *2.4.5*)<br>3. Generally minimal cytologic atypia. High-grade dysplasia may be seen in larger (>1 cm case) examples (*Fig. 2.4.6*)<br>4. 13% cases are associated with invasive carcinoma | 1. Predominantly papillary configuration (*Fig. 2.4.7*)<br>2. Variety of epithelial morphologic patterns have been described (pancreatobiliary, gastric, intestinal, oncocytic) (*Figs. 2.4.8-2.4.11*). They often overlap and do not have clinical implications<br>3. Classified as low-grade or high-grade<br>4. More than half of the cases are associated with an invasive carcinoma (*Fig. 2.4.12*) |
| *Special Studies* | • Immunolabeling: MUC6 positive and MUC2 negative | • Immunolabeling:<br>Biliary type: CK7 and EMA (MUC1) positive<br>Gastric type: MUC5AC diffusely positive, some cases may express MUC6<br>Intestinal type: CK20; CDX2, and MUC2 positive<br>Oncocytic type: EMA (MUC1) positive, negative for MUC6. Fusions in *PRKACA* and *PRKACB* genes |
| *Treatment* | Surgery | Surgery |
| *Prognosis* | If invasive carcinoma is ruled out, patients are cured | Good prognosis if there is no invasive carcinoma |

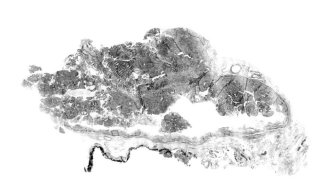

**Figure 2.4.1**    Pyloric gland adenoma. This large example has a sessile configuration.

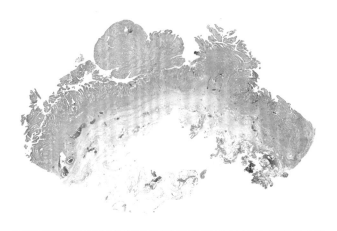

**Figure 2.4.2**    Pyloric gland adenoma. This adenoma has a pedunculated configuration.

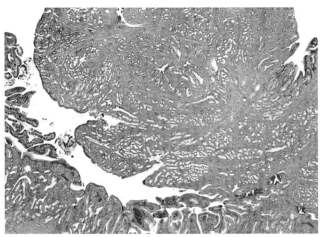

**Figure 2.4.3**    Pyloric gland adenoma. This neoplasm is composed of evenly sized, bland-appearing pyloric-type glands.

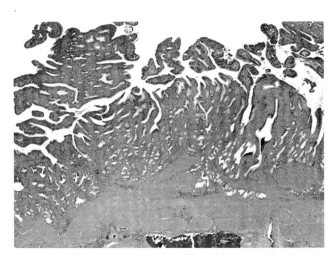

**Figure 2.4.4**    Polypoid pyloric metaplasia. This nodule measures less than 0.5 cm in size and is arising in a background of pyloric metaplasia. It is therefore best classified as nodular pyloric metaplasia, not pyloric gland adenoma.

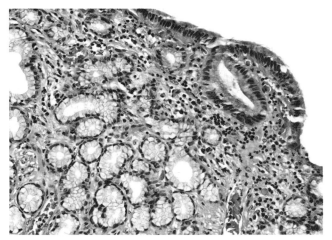

**Figure 2.4.5**    Pyloric gland adenoma. Pyloric type glands are lined by cells with basal nuclei and pale cytoplasm.

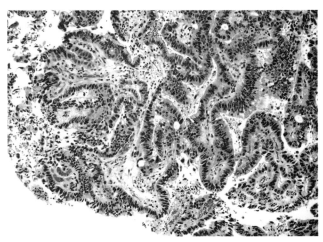

**Figure 2.4.6**    Pyloric gland adenoma. This case has extensive high-grade dysplasia.

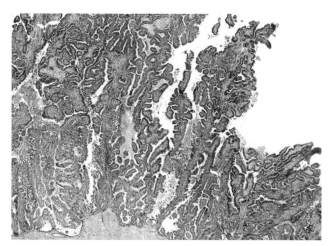

**Figure 2.4.7**    Intracholecystic papillary neoplasm. Note the prominent papillary configuration.

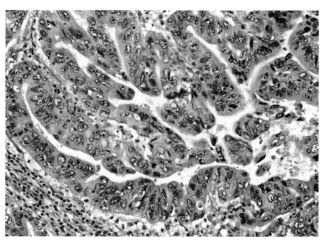

**Figure 2.4.8**    Intracholecystic papillary neoplasm, pancreatobiliary type. This neoplasm is characterized by cuboidal cells with moderate amphophilic cytoplasm and round vesicular nuclei.

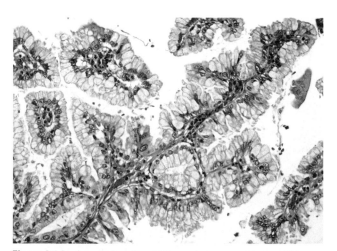

**Figure 2.4.9**    Intracholecystic papillary neoplasm, gastric type. This neoplasm is characterized by low-grade mucinous epithelium with abundant apical cytoplasmic mucin and small basally located nuclei.

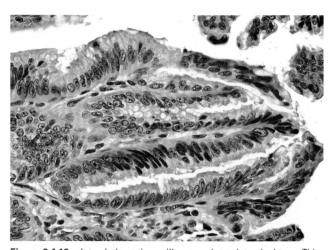

**Figure 2.4.10**    Intracholecystic papillary neoplasm, intestinal type. This neoplasm is characterized by villous papillae with basophilic cytoplasm and elongated nuclei with pseudostratification. Slightly amphophilic apical mucin is characteristic of the intestinal type.

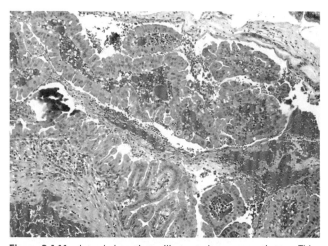

**Figure 2.4.11**    Intracholecystic papillary neoplasm, oncocytic type. This neoplasm is characterized by papillae lined by multiple layers of cells with abundant eosinophilic granular cytoplasm and nuclei with single prominent nucleoli.

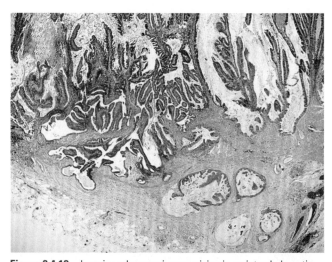

**Figure 2.4.12**    Invasive adenocarcinoma arising in an intracholecystic papillary neoplasm. The neoplastic cells infiltrate into the perimuscular connective tissue.

|  | Luschka Ducts | Adenocarcinoma of Gallbladder |
|---|---|---|
| *Age* | 50–80 y of age | A mean age of 65 y |
| *Location* | The gallbladder fossa adjacent to the liver | Fundus (60%), body (30%), neck (10%) |
| *Symptom* | Incidental finding in gallbladders removed for cholecystitis | Two-thirds of the cases are diagnosed incidentally during or after cholecystectomy, common presentation includes steady abdominal pain and jaundice |
| *Signs* | Ultrasound examination shows cholecystitis characterized by thickened gallbladder wall and pericholecystic fluid | Ultrasound examination shows focal or diffuse mural thickening of the gallbladder and/or an intraluminal mass |
| *Etiology* | Developmental abnormality present within the gallbladder fossa adjacent to the liver | Gallstones. Known association with primary sclerosing cholangitis, pancreatobiliary maljunction, *Salmonella typhi* infection, Lynch syndrome, and familial adenomatous polyposis |
| *Histology* | 1. Present only in adventitia *(Fig. 2.5.1)*<br>2. Lobular or linear architecture<br>3. Concentric fibrosis around glands *(Fig. 2.5.2)*<br>4. Cytology characterized by reactive atypia with inflammation<br>5. Mitoses are rare to none *(Fig. 2.5.3)*<br>6. Perineural and vascular invasion are not seen | 1. Involve the full thickness *(Fig. 2.5.4)*<br>2. Haphazard architecture<br>3. Irregular fibrosis *(Fig. 2.5.5)*<br>4. Nuclear variation (≥4:1) within a single gland *(Fig. 2.5.6)*<br>5. Mitoses are usually present and may be abnormal<br>6. Vascular or perineural invasion may be present *(Fig. 2.5.7)* |
| *Special Studies* | • Intact Smad4 immunolabeling | • Loss of Smad4 immunolabeling in 50% cases |
| *Treatment* | Incidental finding—none needed | Surgery |
| *Prognosis* | Over diagnosis as adenocarcinoma may have serious consequences. They can be a source of bile leak after cholecystectomy; otherwise, excellent prognosis | Overall, 5-y survival rate 10%–20% |

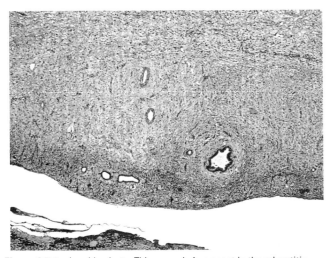

**Figure 2.5.1** Luschka ducts. This example is present in the adventitia without accompanying vessels.

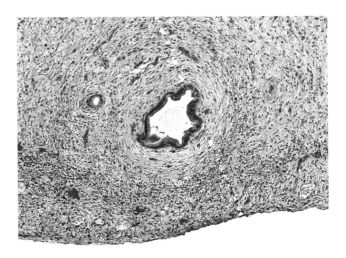

**Figure 2.5.2** Luschka ducts. These benign ducts maintain a lobular architecture. Note the concentric fibrosis around the glands. Higher magnification of Figure 2.5.1.

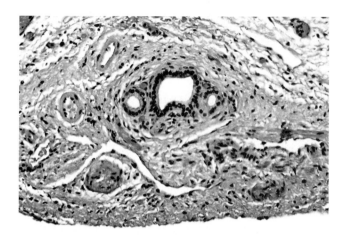

**Figure 2.5.3** Luschka ducts. Cytologic atypia is minimal.

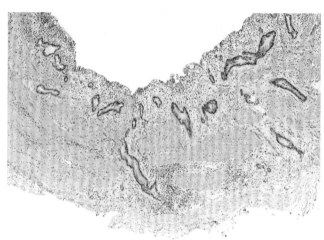

**Figure 2.5.4** Invasive adenocarcinoma. The neoplastic cells involve the full thickness of the gallbladder wall and grow in a haphazard fashion.

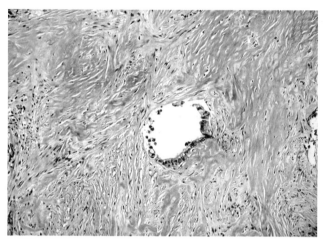

**Figure 2.5.5** Invasive adenocarcinoma. Irregular fibrosis is noted around the invasive carcinoma.

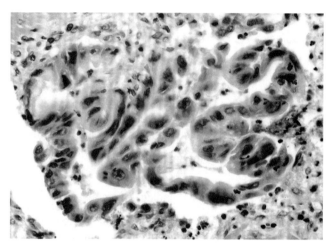

**Figure 2.5.6** Invasive adenocarcinoma. Nuclear variation greater than 4:1 is present in a single gland.

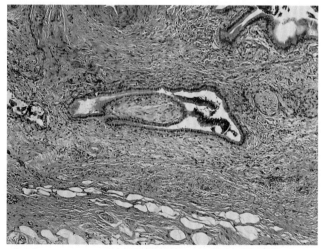

**Figure 2.5.7** Adenocarcinoma. Note the perineural invasion.

| | Extrahepatic Ducts With Reactive Changes | Biliary Intraepithelial Neoplasia (BilIN) |
|---|---|---|
| *Age* | Any age | Elderly |
| *Location* | Anywhere within the bile duct | Anywhere within the bile duct |
| *Symptom* | Incidental finding | Incidental finding |
| *Signs* | None | None |
| *Etiology* | Inflammation | Chronic inflammation |
| *History* | Instrumentation or stent placement | Cholangiocarcinoma, familial adenomatous polyposis, primary sclerosing cholangitis, choledochal cyst, or anomalous union of pancreatobiliary ducts |
| *Histology* | 1. Usually flat *(Fig. 2.6.1)*<br>2. Nuclei are round or oval with smooth nuclear membranes<br>3. Nuclear chromatin is fine and homogeneously distributed *(Fig. 2.6.2)*<br>4. Preserved lobular architecture *(Fig. 2.6.3)*<br>5. Surface maturation present<br>6. Inflammatory cells are present *(Fig. 2.6.4)*<br>7. Involvement of peribiliary glands is infrequent | 1. Lesion can be flat, pseudopapillary or micropapillary<br>2. Hyperchromatic nuclei, high-grade BilIN has irregular nuclei *(Figs. 2.6.5 and 2.6.6)*<br>3. Nuclear stratification, high-grade BilIN has complex nuclear stratification *(Fig. 2.6.7)*<br>4. Increased N:C ratio. High-grade has pleomorphism, and bizarre nuclei *(Fig. 2.6.8)*<br>5. Surface maturation absent<br>6. Inflammatory cells are absent<br>7. Involvement of peribiliary glands is frequent *(Fig. 2.6.9)* |
| *Special Study* | • TP53: negative immunolabeling | • TP53 immunolabeling:<br>Low-grade = negative<br>High-grade = frequently positive<br>*(Fig. 2.6.10)* |
| *Treatment* | Medical or surgical | Resection for high-grade |
| *Prognosis* | Excellent | Most high-grade BilIN is cured by resection |

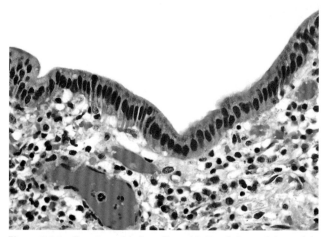

**Figure 2.6.1**    Reactive epithelium. The epithelium is flat and the nuclei are oval with smooth nuclear membranes. The nuclear chromatin is fine and homogeneous.

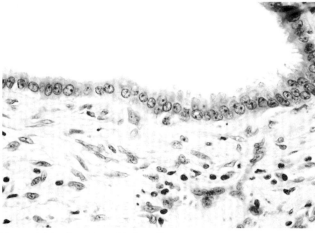

**Figure 2.6.2**    Reactive epithelium. The nuclear chromatin is fine, and the nuclei have small nucleoli.

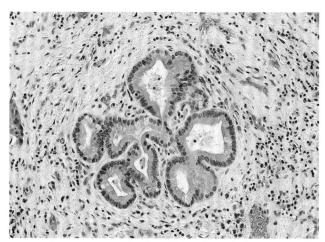

**Figure 2.6.3**    Reactive peribiliary glands. Note the preserved lobular architecture.

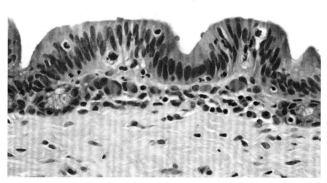

**Figure 2.6.4**    Reactive biliary epithelium. There is focal stratification. Surface maturation and inflammatory cells are present.

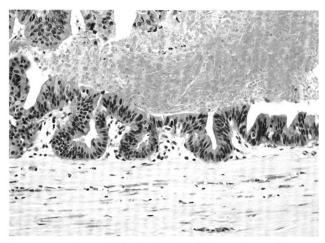

**Figure 2.6.5**    Low-grade dysplasia. This lesion has a micropapillary appearance, and extensive nuclear stratification. The nuclei are hyperchromatic.

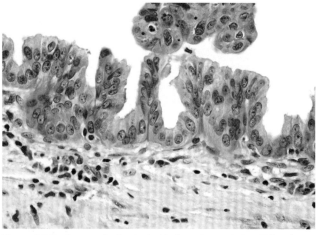

**Figure 2.6.6**    Low-grade dysplasia. Nuclear chromatin is still fine, but extensive nuclear stratification is noted. The nuclear to cytoplasmic (N:C) ratio is slightly increased.

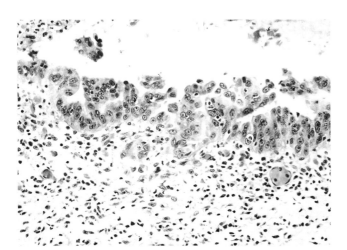

**Figure 2.6.7** High-grade dysplasia. Extensive nuclear stratification is present, and the nuclei have prominent large nucleoli. The N:C ratio is increased and surface maturation is absent.

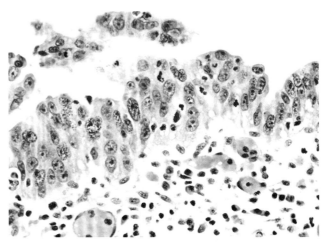

**Figure 2.6.8** High-grade dysplasia. Cellular polarity is distorted. Cytologically malignant features, including severe nuclear membrane irregularities and large nucleoli, are noted.

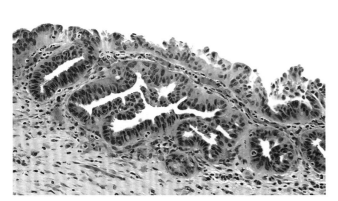

**Figure 2.6.9** High-grade dysplasia. The dysplasia extensively involves peribiliary glands.

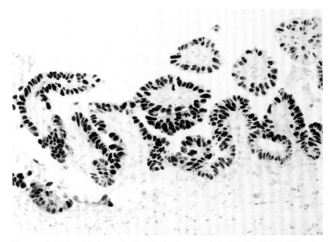

**Figure 2.6.10** High-grade dysplasia. Immunolabeling for TP53 diffusely and strongly labels the dysplastic nuclei.

|  | IgG4-Associated Cholangitis | Primary Sclerosing Cholangitis |
|---|---|---|
| *Age* | Older than 50 y | Younger than 50 y |
| *Location* | Distal or hilar bile ducts | Large bile ducts<br>Small bile duct variant |
| *Symptom* | Obstructive jaundice | Progressive fatigue, pruritus, jaundice |
| *Signs* | Elevated serum IgG4 levels 463 ± 355 (mg/dL)<br>Peripheral eosinophilia 284 ± 219 (/mm³)<br>Segmental stricture visualized by cholangiography | Normal serum IgG levels 32 ± 10 (mg/dL)<br>Normal eosinophil counts 880 ± 104 (/mm³)<br>Beaded appearance in cholangiography<br>Perinuclear antineutrophil cytoplasmic antibodies (pANCA) |
| *Etiology* | Fibroinflammatory condition, often associated with other extrabiliary fibroinflammatory lesions | Unknown, 70% of patient have or will develop inflammatory bowel disease |
| *Histology* | 1. Transmural dense lymphoplasmacytic infiltrate *(Figs. 2.7.1 and 2.7.2)*<br>2. Erosion, lymphoid follicles, and eosinophils are common<br>3. Storiform pattern of fibrosis *(Fig. 2.7.3)*<br>4. Obliterative phlebitis *(Figs. 2.7.4 and 2.7.5)* | 1. Lymphoplasmacytic infiltrate is limited to the lamina propria *(Fig. 2.7.7)*<br>2. Ulcer, erosion, and neutrophilic infiltrate is common *(Figs. 2.7.8 and 2.7.9)*<br>3. Concentric periductal fibrosis around middle to small bile ducts *(Figs. 2.7.10 and 2.7.11)*; fibrous obliterative cholangitis of middle to small bile duct *(Figs. 2.7.12 and 2.7.13)*<br>4. Phlebitis is not seen |
| *Special Studies* | • Immunolabeling:<br>IgG4 positive cells >10/HPF (biopsy)<br>IgG4 positive cells >50/HPF (resection) *(Fig. 2.7.6)* | • Immunolabeling:<br>No increase in IgG4-positive cells<br>• HLA-A1, B8, DR3, DR4, DRW52A |
| *Treatment* | Steroid responsive | No medical treatment<br>Liver transplant for decompensated cirrhosis |
| *Prognosis* | No increased risk for cholangiocarcinoma | Progress to biliary cirrhosis within 10–15 y<br>Increased risk for cholangiocarcinoma |

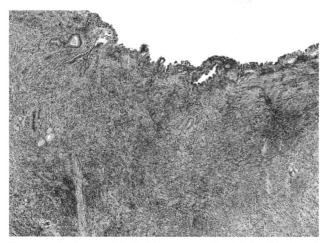

**Figure 2.7.1**  Immunoglobulin G4 (IgG4)–associated cholangitis. Note the dense transmural mononuclear infiltrate involving the bile duct.

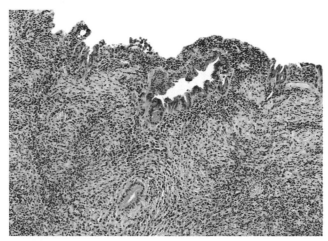

**Figure 2.7.2**  Immunoglobulin G4 (IgG4)–associated cholangitis. The inflammatory cells include lymphocytes, plasma cells, and eosinophils.

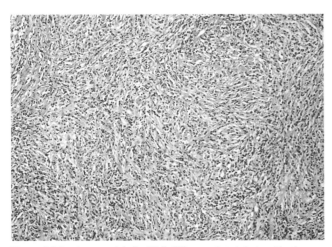

**Figure 2.7.3**    Immunoglobulin G4 (IgG4)–associated cholangitis. A storiform pattern of fibrosis, characterized by loosely arranged whorls of elongated, spindled fibroblast-like cells, is present.

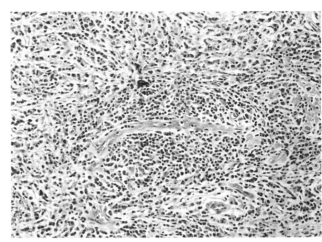

**Figure 2.7.4**    Immunoglobulin G4 (IgG4)–associated cholangitis. Note the obliterative phlebitis in the center of the figure.

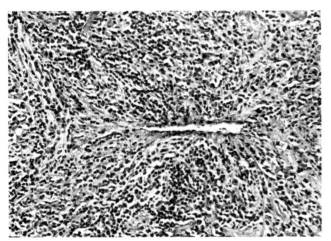

**Figure 2.7.5**    Immunoglobulin G4 (IgG4)–associated cholangitis. A Movat stain highlights an obliterated venule.

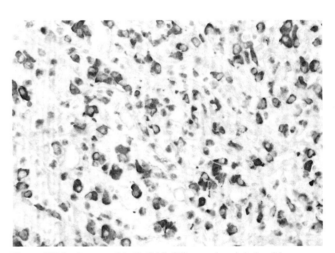

**Figure 2.7.6**    Immunoglobulin G4 (IgG4)–associated cholangitis. Increased numbers of IgG4-positive cells are present. IgG4+/IgG+ plasma cell ratio >40% supports the diagnosis. Diagnostic criteria include >10 IgG4+ cells/high-power field in biopsy specimens and >50 IgG4+ cells/high-power field in resections. (Immunolabeling for IgG4.)

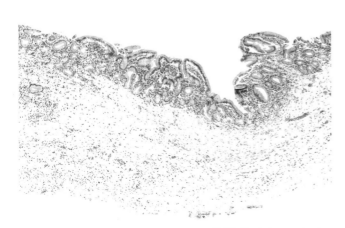

**Figure 2.7.7**    Primary sclerosing cholangitis (PSC). The inflammation is limited in the mucosa.

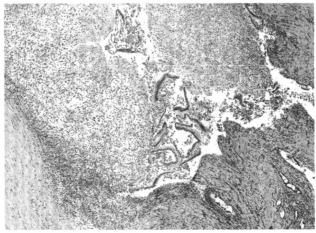

**Figure 2.7.8**    Primary sclerosing cholangitis. This large bile duct is remarkable for epithelial denudation and abscess formation.

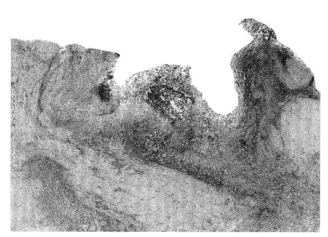

**Figure 2.7.9** Primary sclerosing cholangitis. Epithelial loss in a large bile duct has resulted in a mixture of bile, neutrophils, and granulation tissue along areas of ulceration.

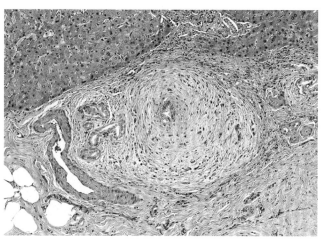

**Figure 2.7.10** Primary sclerosing cholangitis. Note the concentric periductal fibrosis in this medium-sized bile duct.

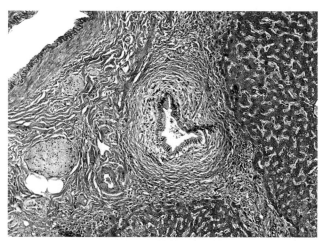

**Figure 2.7.11** Primary sclerosing cholangitis. A trichrome stain highlights concentric fibrosis around a medium-sized bile duct.

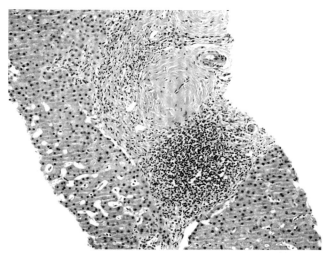

**Figure 2.7.12** Primary sclerosing cholangitis. Fibrous obliteration of small bile duct.

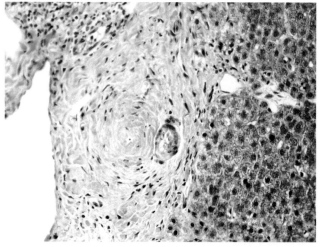

**Figure 2.7.13** Primary sclerosing cholangitis. A trichrome stain highlights fibrous obliteration of a bile duct adjacent to a hepatic artery.

| | Intraductal Papillary Neoplasm of the Bile Duct (IPNB) | Intraductal Metastatic Cancer |
|---|---|---|
| *Age* | 50–70 y of age | Mean age of 55 y |
| *Location* | The prevalent location is highly variable among studies | **Major bile duct in 53% and minor bile duct in 44% for colon cancer** |
| *Symptom* | Abdominal pain, jaundice, cholangitis | Abdominal pain, jaundice, cholangitis |
| *Signs* | Elevated alkaline phosphatase<br>Obstructive lesion in the bile duct by imaging studies | Elevated alkaline phosphatase<br>Obstructive lesion in the bile duct by imaging studies |
| *Etiology* | Most cases are unknown; some cases have history of primary sclerosing cholangitis, hepatolithiasis, liver fluke infection | Metastatic cancer; colon cancer is the most common primary |
| *Histology* | 1. A polypoid mass in a dilated bile duct *(Fig. 2.8.1)*. Lesions <3 mm in height are categorized as micropapillary biliary intraepithelial neoplasia (BilIN) *(Fig. 2.8.2)*<br>2. Papillary structures with fibrovascular cores covered by biliary epithelium *(Fig. 2.8.3)*<br>3. Variety of epithelial morphologic pattern have been described (biliary, gastric, intestinal, oncocytic). These often overlap and have no clinical implication *(Fig. 2.8.4)*<br>4. Classified as low-grade or high-grade | 1. A polypoid mass in a dilated bile duct *(Fig. 2.8.5)*<br>2. Tumor composed plugs of tubular glands in bile duct<br>3. Colonization of bile duct with replacement of the normal biliary epithelium *(Fig. 2.8.6)*. There is often an abrupt transition between the normal epithelium and the cancer<br>4. Various degrees of differentiation depending on primary tumor |
| *Special Studies* | • Immunolabeling:<br>Biliary type: CK7 and EMA (MUC1) positiveGastric type: MUC5AC diffusely positive, some cases may express MUC6<br>Intestinal type: CK20; CDX2, and MUC2 positive<br>Oncocytic type: EMA (MUC1) positive, negative for MUC6, fusions in *PRKACA* and *PRKACB* gene | • Immunolabeling of metastatic colon cancer: CK7 negative *(Fig. 2.8.7)*, CK20 and CDX-2 positive<br>• Various somatic mutations depending on primary tumor |
| *Treatment* | Surgery | Surgery, confirmation of diagnosis generally requires histologic examination of the resected specimen |
| *Prognosis* | Better prognosis than with invasive cholangiocarcinoma | 5-y survival rate is 45% |

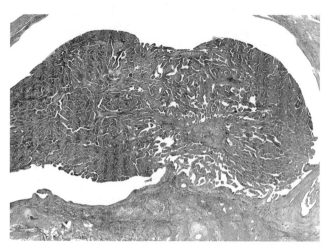

**Figure 2.8.1**    Intraductal papillary neoplasm of the bile duct (IPNB). Note the polypoid mass with a papillary configuration in the bile duct.

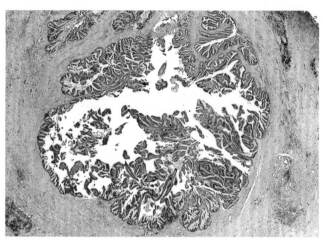

**Figure 2.8.2**    Biliary intraepithelial neoplasia. This neoplasm measures less than 3 mm in height and is therefore best classified as micropapillary biliary intraepithelial neoplasia.

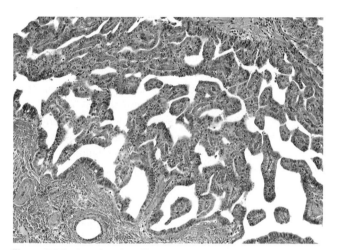

**Figure 2.8.3**    Intraductal papillary neoplasm of the bile duct, pancreatobiliary type. The papillae are lined by biliary type epithelium.

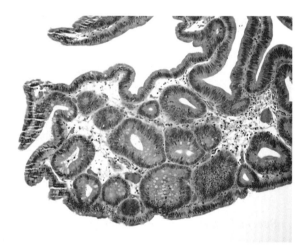

**Figure 2.8.4**    Intraductal papillary neoplasm of the bile duct, intestinal type, with low-grade dysplasia. The neoplastic epithelium has elongated nuclei with pseudostratification. Amphophilic mucin is noted.

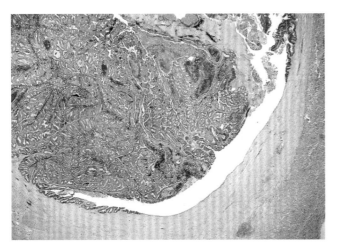

**Figure 2.8.5**   Intraductal metastatic colon cancer. A polypoid mass is noted in a dilated bile duct.

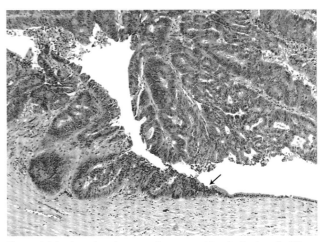

**Figure 2.8.6**   Intraductal metastatic cancer with colonization of a bile duct. An abrupt transition between normal bile duct and the colonized epithelium is noted (*arrow*).

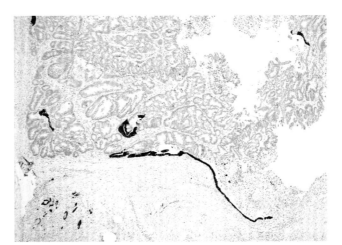

**Figure 2.8.7**   Intraductal metastatic colon cancer. Immunolabeling for cytokeratin 7 is negative, supporting the diagnosis of metastatic colon cancer.

| | Reactive Ampullary Epithelial Changes | Neoplastic Changes Involving Ampullary Epithelium |
|---|---|---|
| Age | Can occur at any age with inciting factors (inflammation, obstruction, stones, etc.) | Wide age range of 32–86 y |
| Location | Anywhere in ampulla and periampullary epithelium | Anywhere in ampulla and periampullary epithelium |
| Symptoms | Related to underlying inciting factors, may be incidental | Usually nonspecific, including abdominal pain and nausea if obstruction from underlying mass lesion |
| Signs | May see ulceration, erosion and other inflammatory changes on endoscopy, no discrete mass lesion | May see ampullary or periampullary mass lesion on imaging |
| Etiology | Inflammation | Multifactorial, dependent on specific neoplasm. May reflect *in situ* dysplasia or colonization by underlying carcinoma |
| Histology | 1. Predominantly involves ampullary surface epithelium. Flat to polypoid<br>2. Round to oval nuclei with smooth nuclear contours and open chromatin. Often single inconspicuous nucleoli *(Figs. 2.9.5-2.9.7)*<br>3. Fairly uniform nuclei. Cells may have a "streaming" appearance with indistinct cell borders but maintenance of polarity *(Figs. 2.9.5-2.9.7)*<br>4. Associated with mixed acute and chronic inflammation, often with ulceration/erosion and granulation tissue *(Figs. 2.9.5-2.9.7)*<br>5. Uniform population of cells across affected areas *(Figs. 2.9.5-2.9.7)* | 1. Involves both ampullary surface and deeper ampullary ducts. May see more complex papillary architecture *(Fig. 2.9.4)*<br>2. Nuclear hyperchromasia, nuclear membrane irregularities, increased nuclear to cytoplasmic ratio *(Figs. 2.9.1-2.9.4)*<br>3. More prominent nuclear pleomorphism, which may be marked. May see loss of polarity with high-grade dysplasia or colonization by carcinoma *(Figs. 2.9.3 and 2.9.4)*<br>4. Inflammation not prominent *(Figs. 2.9.1-2.9.4)*<br>5. Can often appreciate two distinct populations of cells as neoplastic population stands out against adjacent normal *(Fig. 2.9.3)* |
| Special studies | None are consistently helpful | None are consistently helpful |
| Treatment | Medical or surgical depending on inciting cause | Surgical resection when possible |
| Prognosis | Excellent | Dependent on stage of underlying neoplasm |

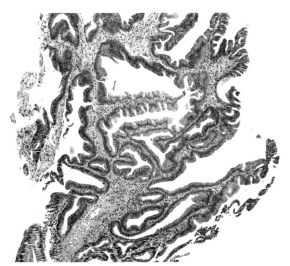

**Figure 2.9.1** Ampullary adenoma. Note the elongated, hyperchromatic nuclei and lack of inflammation.

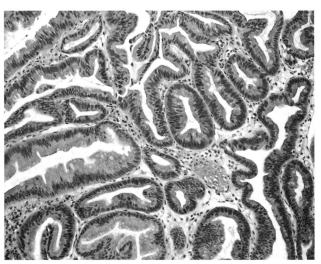

**Figure 2.9.2** Ampullary adenoma. Higher magnification image of different area of adenoma shown in Figure 2.9.1. Note the elongated, hyperchromatic nuclei and lack of inflammation.

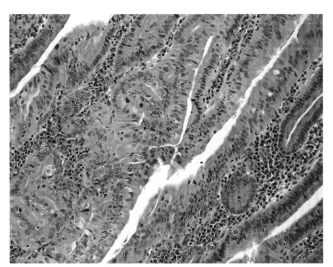

**Figure 2.9.3** High-grade neoplastic epithelium involving ampulla. Note contrast between two cell populations: normal (*lower right*) and neoplastic (*upper left*) with pleomorphism and loss of polarity in the neoplastic cells. Inflammation is not prominent. In this example, the abrupt transition from normal to high-grade cytology suggests the possibility that this represent colonization from an underlying invasive carcinoma.

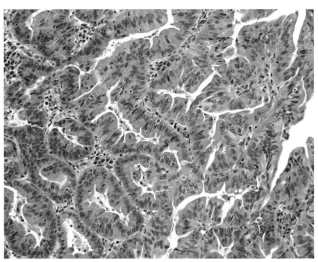

**Figure 2.9.4** High-grade neoplastic epithelium involving ampulla. Note cellular pleomorphism and loss of polarity in the neoplastic cells as well as complex architecture. Inflammation is not prominent. This example could represent either colonization from an underlying invasive carcinoma or *in situ* high-grade dysplasia.

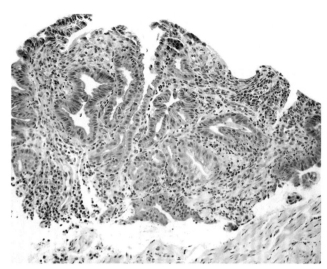

**Figure 2.9.5** Reactive ampullary epithelial changes. Note the uniformity of the cells, smooth nuclear contours and open chromatin. Acute and chronic inflammation are prominent, and there is suggestion of erosion in the top center-right.

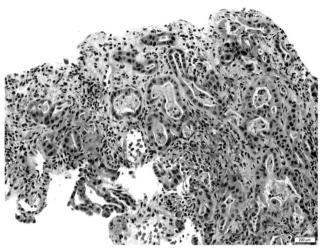

**Figure 2.9.6** Reactive ampullary epithelial changes. Note the uniformity of the cells, smooth nuclear contours and open chromatin. Acute and chronic inflammation are prominent, and there are stromal changes suggestive of prior erosion in the center and lower right.

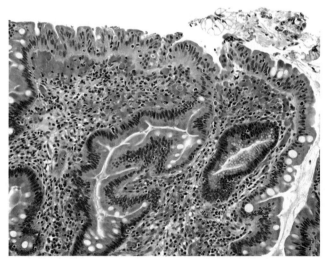

**Figure 2.9.7** Reactive ampullary epithelial changes. This example is more subtle than the changes shown in Figures 2.9.5 and 2.9.6. Note the acute inflammation and irregular surface at the top of the image, consistent with reparative changes.

|  | In Situ Adenomatous Change in Ampulla | Colonization by Underlying Pancreatobiliary Carcinoma |
|---|---|---|
| Age | Wide age range | Seventh and eighth decades of life |
| Location | Anywhere in ampulla and periampullary region | Anywhere in ampulla and periampullary region |
| Symptoms | Usually nonspecific, including abdominal pain and nausea if large adenoma causes obstruction | Epigastric pain, painless jaundice, and nausea |
| Signs | Polypoid/papillary lesion at the ampulla on endoscopy, mass lesion at the ampulla on cross sectional imaging | Weight loss and jaundice. New onset diabetes mellitus in the elderly. 10% develop migratory thrombophlebitis. Mass lesion centered in head of pancreas/periampullary region. Ampulla may appear "prominent" on endoscopy |
| Etiology | May be seen in patients with familial adenomatous polyposis (FAP) | Multiple, including cigarette smoking, obesity, and older age. 10% due to germline mutations in *BRCA2*, *BRCA1*, *PALB2*, *ATM*, *p16/CDKN2A*, *STK11*, *PRSS1*, and in DNA mismatch repair genes (*MLH1*, etc.) |
| Histology | 1. Surface may show complex tubular and tubulovillous projections<br>2. Dysplastic changes transition smoothly and gradually from low-grade to high-grade (*Figs. 2.10.1* and *2.10.2*)<br>3. May show intestinal or pancreatobiliary differentiation | 1. Ampullary surface usually flat unless colonization is extensive<br>2. Abrupt transition from normal/reactive epithelium to high-grade cytology (*Figs. 2.10.3-2.10.6*)<br>3. Pancreatobiliary differentiation (cuboidal nuclei, abundant eosinophilic cytoplasm often with prominent intracellular mucin) |
| Special studies | Immunolabeling with antibodies to Smad4 will show retention of labeling in dysplastic cells | Immunolabeling with antibodies to Smad4 will show loss of staining in colonizing carcinoma in approximately 60% of cases (*Fig. 2.10.7*) |
| Treatment | Surgical resection | Surgical resection for low-stage disease; chemotherapy or combined chemoradiation for unresectable and locally advanced disease. Neoadjuvant therapy is becoming more common even for resectable and for borderline resectable disease |
| Prognosis | Excellent with complete resection and no associated invasive component, can sometimes see recurrence | 9% 5-y survival |

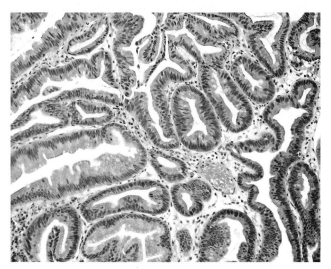

**Figure 2.10.1**    Ampullary adenoma. Note uniform, low-grade dysplasia.

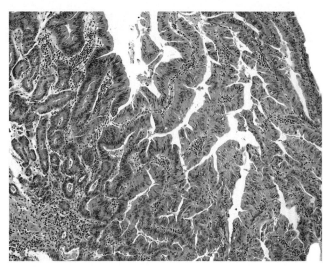

**Figure 2.10.2**    Ampullary adenoma. This example shows a smooth transition from low-grade dysplasia on the left to high-grade dysplasia on the right.

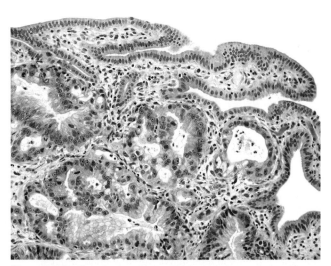

**Figure 2.10.3**    Colonization of ampulla by underlying carcinoma. Note the abrupt transition from normal epithelium (*top and right*) to the high-grade neoplastic epithelium on the left, center, and bottom of the field.

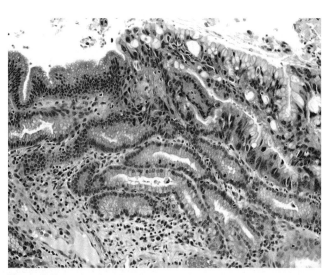

**Figure 2.10.4**    Colonization of ampulla by underlying carcinoma. In this example, high-grade carcinoma colonizes the surface on the top right with an abrupt transition to normal on the left and bottom of the field.

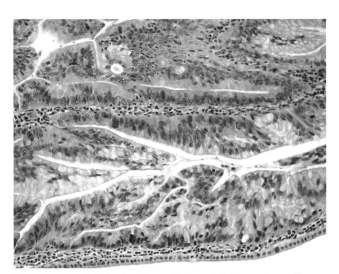

**Figure 2.10.5**   Colonization of ampulla by underlying carcinoma. Note the focal normal epithelium at the bottom of the field.

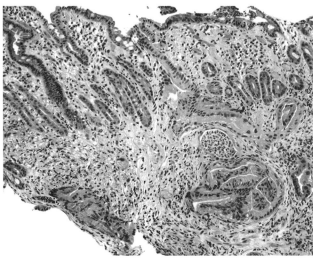

**Figure 2.10.6**   Colonization of ampulla by underlying carcinoma. In this example, normal epithelium is present at the top of the field and a second population of atypical cells with abundant eosinophilic cytoplasm and hyperchromatic nuclei extends up the center of the field and joins with the normal surface. A few atypical single cells in the center left suggest an invasive component. See Smad4 immunolabeling in Figure 2.10.7.

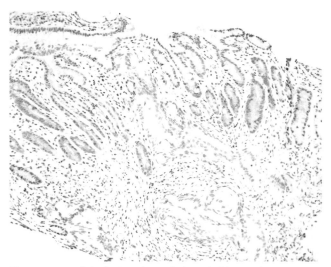

**Figure 2.10.7**   Colonization of ampulla by underlying carcinoma. Immunolabeling for Smad4 in the example shown in Figure 2.10.6 shows loss in the colonizing carcinoma.

| | Ampullary Tubular Adenoma | Intra-Ampullary Papillary-Tubular Neoplasm (IAPN) |
|---|---|---|
| *Age* | Age range 32–86 y | Mean age 64 y, range 27–85 |
| *Location* | Periampullary and/or intra-ampullary region | Intra-ampullary, including intra-ampullary portions of common bile duct and main pancreatic duct |
| *Symptoms* | Asymptomatic, or nonspecific obstructive symptoms | Asymptomatic, or nonspecific obstructive symptoms |
| *Signs* | Polypoid lesion on endoscopy, mass lesion on cross-sectional imaging, involving ampulla/periampullary region | Polypoid/papillary lesion on endoscopy, mass lesion on cross-sectional imaging, centered deep in ampulla |
| *Etiology* | May be seen in patients with familial adenomatous polyposis (FAP) | Unknown |
| *Histology* | 1. Polypoid lesion involving ampulla/periampulla<br>2. Tubular, villous or tubulovillous architecture *(Fig. 2.11.1)*<br>3. Intestinal differentiation *(Fig. 2.11.1)* | 1. Exophytic polypoid or papillary mass within ampullary lumen, site is essential to diagnosis *(Fig. 2.11.2)*<br>2. Mixed papillary and tubular architecture *(Figs. 2.11.2-2.11.5)*<br>3. Intestinal or pancreatobiliary differentiation. Almost half of cases show mixed differentiation *(Figs. 2.11.2-2.11.5)* |
| *Special studies* | None | None |
| *Treatment* | Surgical or endoscopic resection | Surgical or endoscopic resection |
| *Prognosis* | Excellent with complete resection and no associated invasive component, can sometimes see recurrence | Excellent with complete resection and no associated invasive component, can sometimes see recurrence |

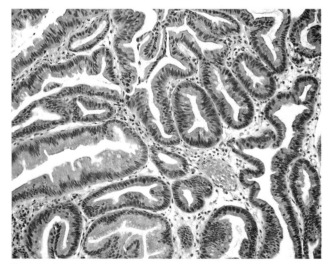

**Figure 2.11.1**   Ampullary tubular adenoma. Note tubular architecture and elongated, "cigar-shaped" nuclei consistent with intestinal differentiation.

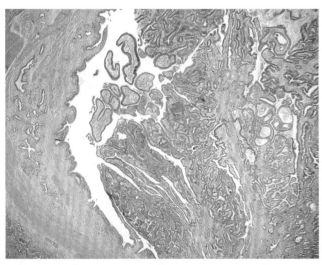

**Figure 2.11.2**   Intra-ampullary papillary-tubular neoplasm. This example shows a complex papillary lesion centered deep in the ampullary channel.

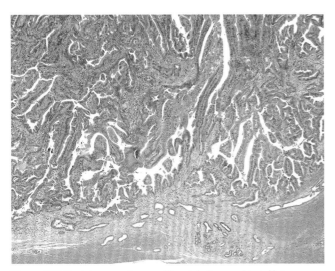

**Figure 2.11.3**   Intra-ampullary papillary-tubular neoplasm. Note the mixed tubular and papillary architecture with predominantly pancreatobiliary differentiation.

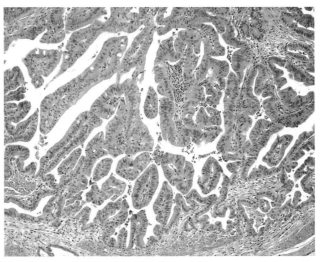

**Figure 2.11.4**   Intra-ampullary papillary-tubular neoplasm. Higher magnification image of the neoplasm shown in Figure 2.11.3.

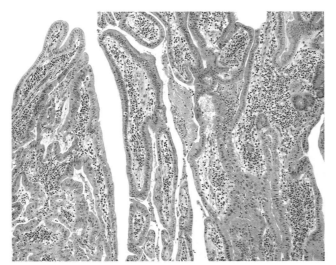

**Figure 2.11.5**   Intra-ampullary papillary-tubular neoplasm. Note the elongated papillary architecture and pancreatobiliary differentiation.

| | Well-Differentiated Ampullary Neuroendocrine Tumor | Gangliocytic Paraganglioma |
|---|---|---|
| *Age* | Adults in the sixth decade of life | Mean age 52 y, range 15–84 |
| *Location* | Ampulla, periampullary region, distal duodenum | Periampullary region and second portion of duodenum |
| *Symptoms* | Asymptomatic, or nonspecific obstructive symptoms, rarely carcinoid syndrome | Asymptomatic, or may present with gastrointestinal bleeding or abdominal pain |
| *Signs* | Polypoid lesion on endoscopy, mass lesion on cross-sectional imaging, involving ampulla/periampullary region | Polypoid lesion on endoscopy, mass lesion on cross-sectional imaging, involving ampulla/periampullary region or duodenum |
| *Etiology* | May be seen in patients with neurofibromatosis (somatostatinomas) or multiple neuroendocrine neoplasia, Type 1 (MEN1) (duodenal, often gastrinomas) | Unknown |
| *Histology* | 1. Polypoid submucosal lesion<br>2. Cellular, monomorphic low-power appearance. Neoplastic cells form nests and cords. Cells are separated by thin-walled vessels. Can see rosettes or acini *(Fig. 2.12.1)*<br>3. Rounded or polygonal cells with abundant amphophilic cytoplasm. Low nuclear to cytoplasmic ratio. Uniform nuclei with "salt and pepper" chromatin. Inconspicuous nucleoli *(Fig. 2.12.1)*<br>4. Mitotic rate/proliferative index defines grade (<2 per 10 HPF or Ki67 <3%, grade 1; 2–20 per 10 HPF or Ki67 3%–20%, grade 2; >20 per 10 HPF or Ki67 >20%, grade 3), but even grade 3 typically have Ki67 labeling index <55% | 1. Unencapsulated lesion centered in the submucosa<br>2. Triphasic growth pattern comprised of epithelioid cells, spindle cells (Schwannian stroma) and ganglion cells. Epithelioid cells may show nested and/or trabecular architecture *(Figs. 2.12.2-2.12.6 and 2.12.8)*<br>3. Cells in epithelioid regions resemble well-differentiated neuroendocrine tumor, distinction on biopsy may be difficult if other components are not sampled *(Fig. 2.12.2)*<br>4. No grading system |
| *Special studies* | • Immunolabel with antibodies to cytokeratin<br>• Diffusely immunolabel with antibodies to synaptophysin and chromogranin<br>• No immunolabeling with antibodies to S100 | • Epithelioid cells will immunolabel with antibodies to cytokeratin<br>• Epithelioid cells and ganglion cells will immunolabel with antibodies to synaptophysin and chromogranin *(Fig. 2.12.7)*<br>• Ganglion cells and spindle cells (Schwannian stroma) will immunolabel with antibodies to S100 *(Fig. 2.12.9)* |
| *Treatment* | Surgical or endoscopic resection | Surgical or endoscopic resection |
| *Prognosis* | Malignant. Prognosis depends on grade (proliferation rate) and stage | Good, usually indolent behavior. Metastases are extremely rare, but can recur if incompletely resected |

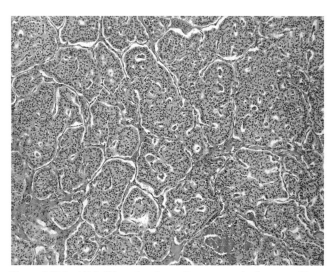

**Figure 2.12.1**    Well-differentiated ampullary neuroendocrine tumor. Note uniform population of epithelioid cells with prominent nested architecture.

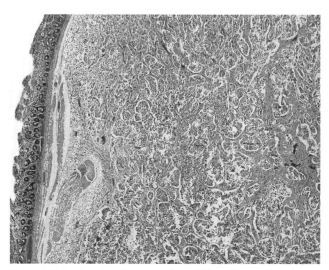

**Figure 2.12.2**    Gangliocytic paraganglioma. This field predominantly shows the epithelioid component, but spindled (Schwannian) stroma is evident between the nests, most prominently on the right side of the image.

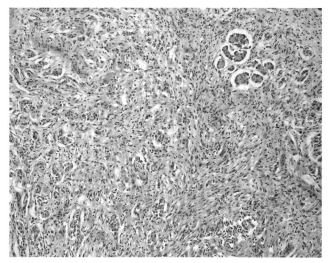

**Figure 2.12.3**    Gangliocytic paraganglioma. This example shows all three components of the triphasic morphology: epithelioid, spindled, and ganglionic.

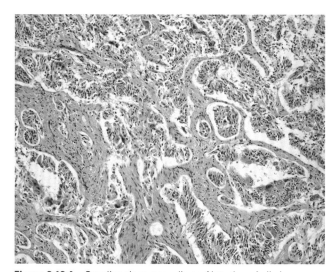

**Figure 2.12.4**    Gangliocytic paraganglioma. Note the spindled (Schwannian stroma) coursing between nests of epithelioid cells.

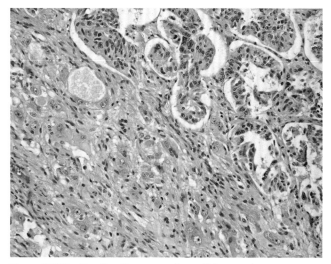

**Figure 2.12.5**    Gangliocytic paraganglioma. This example more prominently highlights the ganglionic component (*left and center bottom*).

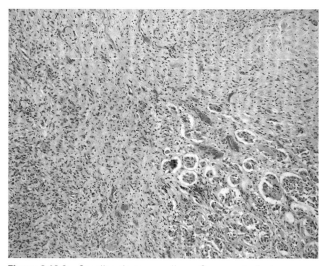

**Figure 2.12.6**    Gangliocytic paraganglioma. See synaptophysin immunolabeling in Figure 2.12.7.

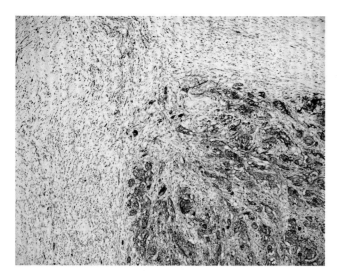

**Figure 2.12.7** Gangliocytic paraganglioma. Synaptophysin immunolabeling highlights the epithelioid and ganglionic components.

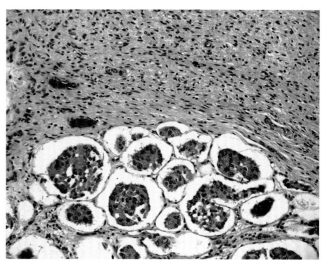

**Figure 2.12.8** Gangliocytic paraganglioma. See S100 immunolabeling in Figure 2.12.9.

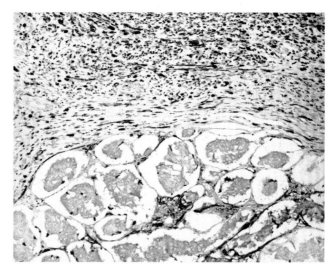

**Figure 2.12.9** Gangliocytic paraganglioma. S100 immunolabeling highlights the spindled (Schwannian) stroma.

## SUGGESTED READINGS

**Chapters 2.1-2.8**

Adsay V, Jang KT, Roa JC, et al. Intracholecystic papillary-tubular neoplasms (ICPN) of the gallbladder (neoplastic polyps, adenomas, and papillary neoplasms that are ≥1.0 cm): clinicopathologic and immunohistochemical analysis of 123 cases. *Am J Surg Pathol.* September 2012;36(9):1279-1301.

Albores-Saavedra J, Chablé-Montero F, González-Romo MA, Ramírez Jaramillo M, Henson DE. Adenomas of the gallbladder. Morphologic features, expression of gastric and intestinal mucins, and incidence of high-grade dysplasia/carcinoma in situ and invasive carcinoma. *Hum Pathol.* September 2012;43(9):1506-1513.

Albores-Saavedra J, Henson DE, Klimstra DS. *Tumor of the Gallbladder, Extrahepatic Bile Ducts, and Vaterian System. AFIP Atlas of Tumor Pathology Series 4;* 2017.

Basturk O, Hong SM, Wood LD, et al. A revised classification system and recommendations from the Baltimore consensus meeting for neoplastic precursor lesions in the pancreas. *Am J Surg Pathol.* December 2015;39(12):1730-1741.

Deshpande V, Zen Y, Chan JK, et al. Consensus statement on the pathology of IgG4-related disease. *Mod Pathol.* September 2012;25(9):1181-1192. doi:10.1038/modpathol.2012.72. PMID: 22596100.

Jessurun J, Pambuccian S. Infectious and inflammatory disorders of the gallbladder and extrahepatic biliary tract. In: Odxe RD, Goldblum JR, eds. *Surgical Pathology of the Gastrointestinal Tract, Liver, Biliary Tract and Pancreas.* 3rd ed. Elsevier Saunders; 2014.

Klimstra DS, Lam AK, Paradis V, Schirmacher P. Tumours of the gallbladder and extrahepatic bile ducts. In: Bosman FT, Carneiro F, Hruban RH, Theise ND, eds. *WHO Classification of Tumors of the Digestive System,* Lyon: IARC Press; 2019.

Nishino T, Oyama H, Hashimoto E, et al. Clinicopathological differentiation between sclerosing cholangitis with autoimmune pancreatitis and primary sclerosing cholangitis. *J Gastroenterol.* July 2007;42(7):550-559.

Ragazzi M, Carbonara C, Rosai J. Nonneoplastic signet-ring cells in the gallbladder and uterine cervix. A potential source of overdiagnosis. *Hum Pathol.* March 2009;40(3):326-331.

Singhi AD, Wood LD, Parks E, et al. Recurrent rearrangements in PRKACA and PRKACB in intraductal oncocytic papillary neoplasms of the pancreas and bile duct. *Gastroenterology.* February 2020;158(3):573-582.

Singhi AD, Adsay NV, Swierczynski SL, et al. Hyperplastic Luschka ducts: a mimic of adenocarcinoma in the gallbladder fossa. *Am J Surg Pathol.* 2011;35(6):883-890.

Zen Y, Aishima S, Ajioka Y, et al. Proposal of histological criteria for intraepithelial atypical/proliferative biliary epithelial lesions of the bile duct in hepatolithiasis with respect to cholangiocarcinoma: preliminary report based on interobserver agreement. *Pathol Int.* April 2005;55(4):180-188. doi:10.1111/j.1440-1827.2005.01816.x. PMID: 15826244.

**Chapters 2.9-2.12**

Klimstra DS, Nagtegaal ID, Rugge M, Salto-Tellez M. Tumors of the small intestine and ampulla. In: Bosman FT, Carneiro F, Hruban RH, Theise ND, eds. *World Health Organization Classification of Tumours,* 5th ed.: Digestive System Tumours. Lyon: IARC Press; 2019:111-134.

Ohike N, Kim GE, Tajiri T, et al. Intra-ampullary papillary-tubular neoplasm (IAPN): characterization of tumoral intraepithelial neoplasia occurring within the ampulla: a clinicopathologic analysis of 82 cases. *Am J Surg Pathol.* 2010;34:1731-1748.

Adsay V, Ohike N, Tajiri T, et al. Ampullary region carcinomas: definition and site specific classification with delineation of four clinicopathologically and prognostically distinct subsets in an analysis of 249 cases. *Am J Surg Pathol.* 2012;36:1592-1608.

# INDEX